Back to the Basics

Strength & Conditioning Manual

By Coach Anthony Stone &
Coach Cody Casazza, NCSF Certified Strength Coach

www.CoachStoneFootball.com

ISBN-13: 9798580759364

Printed in the United States of America & Independently published.

All of the exercises, lifts, drills, and teaching strategies or techniques included in this book are only suggestions for working and playing with ages 12 & up. When selecting lifts, exercises, or games for your own sports program or school, you may need to change or modify them to make them developmentally appropriate for your specific situation, including your facilities, equipment, and the players you are working with. Use all suggestions offered at your own risk, and at your own discretion, making sure to take into account all necessary precautions. The authors shall have neither liability nor responsibility in the case of injury to any person using or participating in any of the exercises, lifts, drills, skills, or techniques contained in this book.

Table of Contents

Preface
Coach Stone

This book is dedicated to my lovely wife Kara and our five children: Jade, Anthony Jr., Alexis, Chloe, and Sage, for their continued love and support. You give me strength and confidence by always coming to my football games, allowing me to coach in town and across the world, for always believing in me, and being my number one fans. You are my world!

I also want to thank all of the Coaches who encouraged me along the way, from when I was a student-athlete to my colleagues today. I would not be where I am without your support and direction. To ALL the Youth Coaches: I want to thank you for stepping up and volunteering your time to coach our **Future.** You are laying a foundation and setting an example of what a leader should be.

Thank you Coach Cody Casazza for co-authoring this manual with me. I have enjoyed all of our long conversations about strength & conditioning, football, and life. It has been an honor to watch you grow over the years into the man you have become. I look forward to many more adventures with you.

Jessica Johnson, you have been there from the start by designing my Back to the Basics logo and every book cover. Thank You! I highly recommend contacting her at jess.renee@live.com to have her help you design your logo. Like her on Facebook at: ***@JessicaReneeDesign***

#HCC #FootballFamily

Coach Casazza

I have been blessed to learn from many great men through this game, about life, football, and being a man. So, I would like to say thank you to: Anthony Stone, Rick Schmitz, Jay Emmons, Jason Jefferson, and Vic Wallace. There are many more, however, the men listed above have had an extraordinary impact on me, and I owe a lot of who I am to them. I also owe an insurmountable debt to my wife, Rachel. Thank you for unconditional support and moving across the country so I can continue to learn and grow my passion. Last, I would like to thank my Mom and Grandfather for raising me with a work ethic great enough to handle the sport and all that comes with it.

Life is like football, you will never succeed on your own, you must be able to rely on others and have others rely on you!

I would like to also give a shout out to Amber and Pierre Suter of Spring Hill Fitness located in Spring Hill, TN for allowing me to use their amazing facility in order to complete this book. You guys rock!

SPRING HILL FITNESS

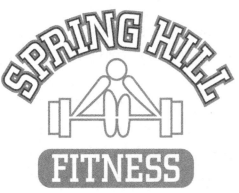

Coach Stone's Coaching Experience

I am humbled and grateful for the coaching opportunities I have had over the years. If you know me, you know #ILOVEFOOTBALL! Coaching football is a passion of mine that supersedes any job title. The one experience that always stands out is being turned down for a Head Coach position a long time ago. I was told that my experience was great, but the reason they did not select me as their High School Head Coach was because I did not have enough experience as a Head Coach. My reply to the athletic director was, "Well, I can't get experience unless someone gives me the opportunity." After that, I came to realize that as coaches we are not defined by a title but by how much our players grow. *Coaching Tip*: Do not get discouraged; stay focused on your why; love what you do; and continually challenge yourself to grow.

Coach Casazza's Coaching Experience

Football has opened many doors in my life, and is providing a never ending purpose to help young men develop a work ethic great enough to achieve any goal or obstacle they may encounter.

I am going into my fifth year coaching football. I've spent 4 seasons as a Defensive Line Coach, 1 year as a Defensive Coordinator, and 2 seasons as the Strength and Conditioning Coordinator. I am a Board Certified Strength and Conditioning Coach through the National Council of Strength & Fitness. In a short time coaching, I have learned a great deal, I have been lucky enough to be around a lot of great coaches to learn from and I've been around some not so great coaches to learn what not to do as well. I am constantly looking for growth opportunities, everything from AFCA National Conventions, Glazier Clinics, YouTube Clinics, & social media. As coaches we are doing the kids and the game a disservice if we pass on opportunities to grow.

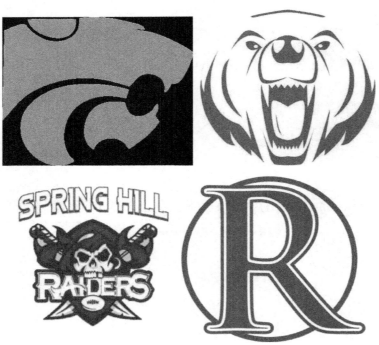

Chapter 1:
Coach Stone's Back to the Basics Model

Introduction

This chapter lays a foundation specific to the content within this *Strength & Conditioning Manual*. It includes a total breakdown from point A to point Z - from Template of an Exercise© to muscles, terminology and much more.

The content within this manual only applies to strength and conditioning exercises for ages 12 & up. The most important thing to remember when coaching strength and conditioning within certain age groups is to include everyone and make it FUN! As a coach it is important to remember the following: never pressure them or push them so hard that they get hurt and then start disliking strength and conditioning.

This *Strength & Conditioning Manual* includes exercises that are specific for ALL Sports.

Coaching Tip:

- Be sure to use or adjust the exercises to meet the age group and special needs of your team as well as the kind of strength & conditioning program you implement. We kept the exercises straightforward and to the point by using our Template of an Exercise©.

The Template of an Exercise© will include:

The Exercise:
Purpose:
Applies to the following Sport(s):
Applies to the following Position(s):
Equipment:
Spotter:
Technique:
Pictures / CCC / CSC Youtube Channel:
Max Out Procedure:
Alternated Lifts / Modification:

The Exercise: This is the name of the exercise the athlete is doing.

Purpose: What. Why? Where. Detailed explanation of the lift and its importance.

Applies to the following Sport(s): What sport(s) this exercise benefits.

Applies to the following Position(s): What position(s) this exercise benefits.

Equipment: The items that should be standard in a weight facility. These will be needed to perform the lifts successfully and safely.

Spotter: Safety first. This is to make sure you are safe when doing these exercises. (Yes, a spotter is needed) (No, a spotter is not needed).

Technique: This is the step by step process on how any specific lift should be performed correctly. Proper technique is needed in order for the athlete to remain healthy, prevent future injury, and transfer to the field of play.

Pictures / CCC / CSC Youtube Channel: Look at pictures from Coach Casazza's YouTube Channel (subscribe NOW): Coach Casazza Strength & Conditioning

Max Out Procedure: This is the process in which the coaching staff / strength staff will take in order to record official max numbers. Max numbers are needed in order to effectively manage a training program.

Alternated Lifts / Modification: This is a list of alternated lifts and different ways you can change the exercises to be more successful. These will be useful if a player has an injury, or condition that does not allow for normal lifting.

Coach Stone Football: Back to the Basics

NOTE: *If you are looking for drills specific to football, you can find them in Coach Stone's Football Drill Manual series which is available on Amazon: Back to the Basics: Football Drill Manual (Green Book) and Volumes I-V.*

The purpose of my company, Coach Stone Football, is to "Instill confidence by laying a foundation one drill at a time." When I first created Coach Stone Football it was clear to me that as coaches, we need to stop trying to find the "next best thing" to make our players better at running, blocking, catching, and tackling, and focus on going Back to the Basics to lay a foundation that instills confidence. This purpose carries over to ALL sports.

Everything I offer is customized to meet the needs of your organization. Go to my website for more information, testimonials, or to contact me with any questions:

Website: www.CoachStoneFootball.com
Email: CoachStoneUSA@gmail.com
Twitter: @Coach_Stone_MT
YouTube Channel: Coach Stone Football: Back to the Basics

Muscles

The human body consists of around 640 skeletal muscles. In Coach Stone's physical education class, he tells his students that the human body is like a car. You need to take care of it or it will break down. The most important muscle of the body is the heart; the heart of the car is its engine. If your heart or the engine isn't working then you are not going to be able to move or run.

There are three main types of muscles in the human body: cardiac, skeletal, and smooth.

- **Cardiac**: These muscles are the ones that are found inside the walls of the heart.

- **Skeletal:** These are the muscles attached to the bones.

- **Smooth**: These muscles are the ones inside the wall of internal organs.

Anterior Muscle Groups

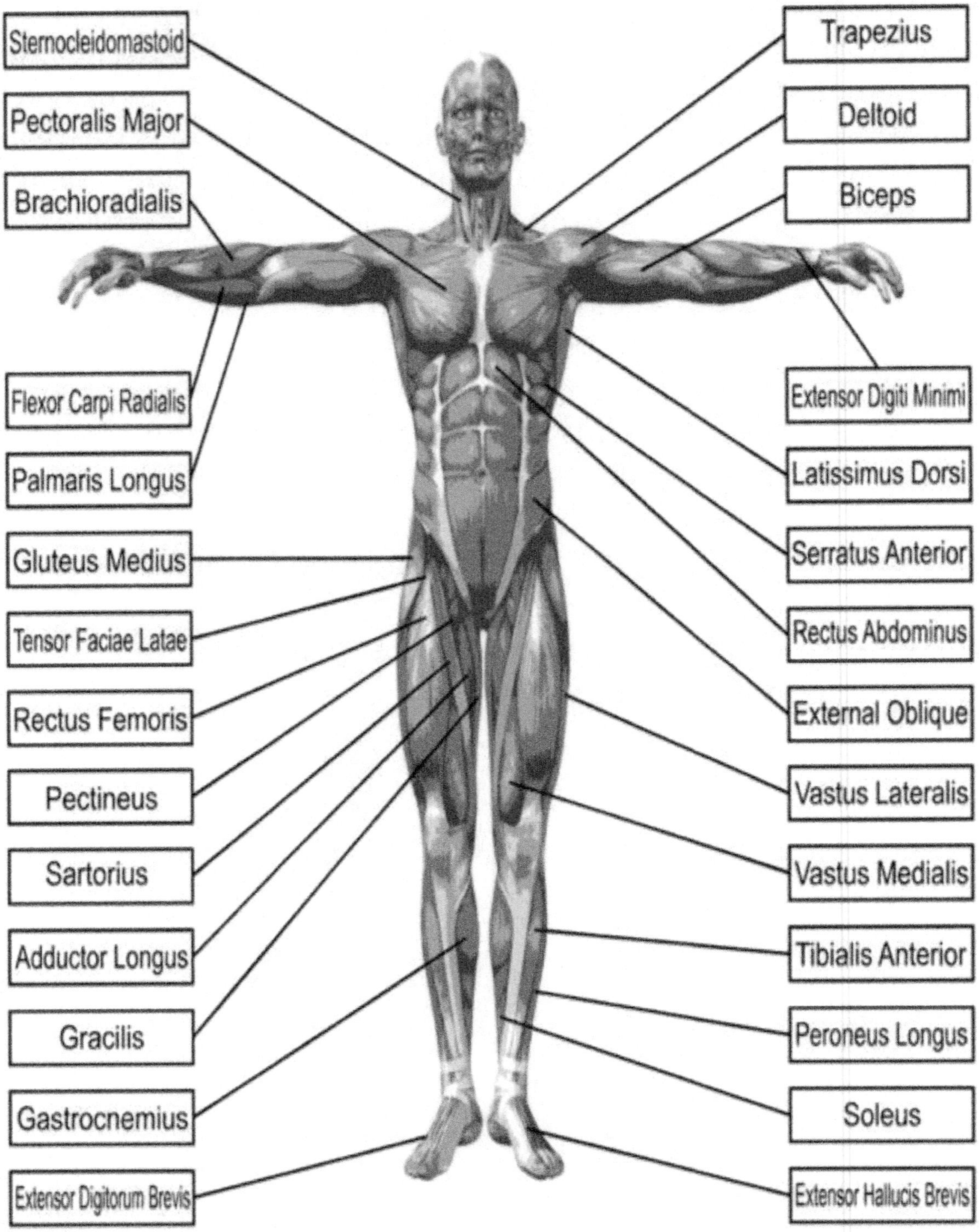
Sternocleidomastoid
Pectoralis Major
Brachioradialis
Flexor Carpi Radialis
Palmaris Longus
Gluteus Medius
Tensor Faciae Latae
Rectus Femoris
Pectineus
Sartorius
Adductor Longus
Gracilis
Gastrocnemius
Extensor Digitorum Brevis
Trapezius
Deltoid
Biceps
Extensor Digiti Minimi
Latissimus Dorsi
Serratus Anterior
Rectus Abdominus
External Oblique
Vastus Lateralis
Vastus Medialis
Tibialis Anterior
Peroneus Longus
Soleus
Extensor Hallucis Brevis

Posterior Muscle Groups

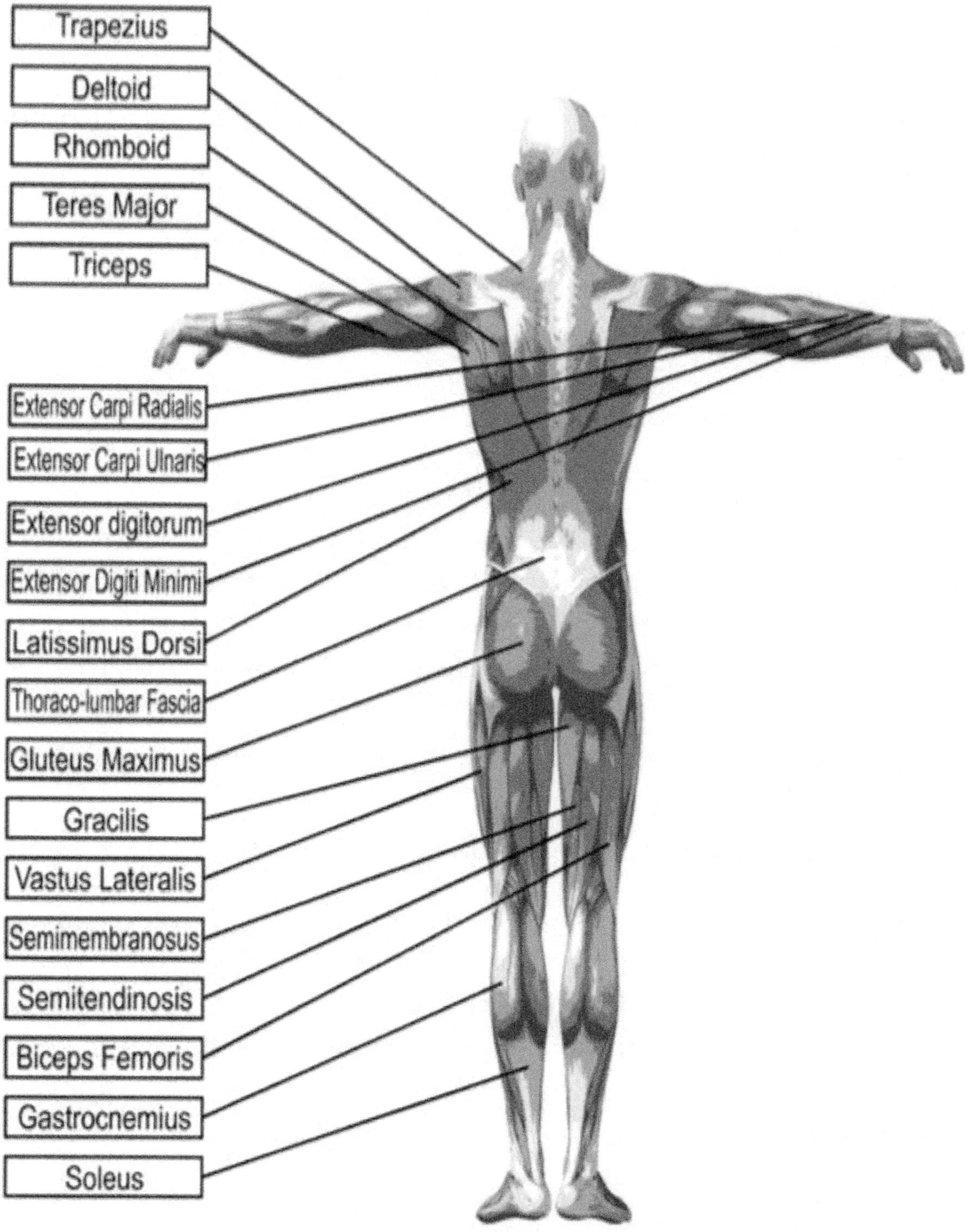
Trapezius
Deltoid
Rhomboid
Teres Major
Triceps
Extensor Carpi Radialis
Extensor Carpi Ulnaris
Extensor digitorum
Extensor Digiti Minimi
Latissimus Dorsi
Thoraco-lumbar Fascia
Gluteus Maximus
Gracilis
Vastus Lateralis
Semimembranosus
Semitendinosis
Biceps Femoris
Gastrocnemius
Soleus

Athletics vs Fitness

In some dictionaries it reads that **athletics** is "physical activities such as sports and games that require stamina, fitness, and skill." Whereas, **Fitness** is "the condition of being fit, suitable or appropriate." Training to be "fit" and training to be an "athlete" are two very different goals.

If you were to walk into your average gym or sports club you would see a lot of people working out and aiming to achieve some level of fitness. Those workouts for the most part will consist of a lot of single joint, isolated movements aimed towards toning a specified target of muscles.

Walking into a sport team's weight session will be a completely different beast, as it should be. The design of the program is built to improve athletic performance (power, strength, speed, agility, quickness, etc.). It will consist of compound movements, several different levels of tempo, in most cases a lot of weight being used in explosive movements, sprinting, jumping, and most importantly, competition.

Athletes come in All Sizes Today

Athletes today, no matter what sport you play or played, have changed over the years. Did you know, in the 1970s there was only one NFL player that weighed 300 or more. Today, the NFL average weight for an offensive lineman is over 300 pounds and also the defensive tackles. But what's funny is they are considered athletic but they might not have good fitness levels and according to their BMI they would be labeled as obese.

Attributes of an Athletic Body

Depending what sport an athlete is training for, the athlete's body should be trained for strength, power, speed, agility, quickness, and endurance. An athlete's body that is built for an endurance sport, such as marathon racing, may be severely limited when it comes to strength, power, speed, and quickness -- particularly in the upper body, or even flexibility. While some sports, such as gymnastics may require the athlete to be proficient in most if not all of these attributes, others have more very specific requirements and therefore the body type of the athlete performing them may not be as well-rounded. An athlete's body type more often than not reflects the most commonly relied upon skills needed for their sport -- for example, again think of a sumo wrestler. A body that is fit should meet specific criteria. These components are:

- **Being Flexible**
- **Cardiovascular Fitness**
- **Body Composition**
- **Muscular Strength**
- **Muscular Endurance**

When determining what position an athlete should play, it is important to factor in an athlete's body type/size not just if they are athletic or not. Because every sport has different criteria to meet in order to be successful. Training requirements for one sport is different than other sports. If you train for one specific sport you should be athletic in that one sport. If the player is a multi-sport athlete it is important to make specific adjustments to their plan that benefits as a "whole" athlete, not a "sport specific" athlete.

Components For Athletic Performance

POWER - (Force x Distance) / Time = Power

This is going to be the biggest distinction between fitness training and athletic development, because this is where the training is going to be different, and unique for athletes.

So, how does being "strong" differ from being "powerful"? The biggest difference is the speed at which the weight is moved. The best example of this is powerlifters, ironically the term "power" is used to describe their craft, when in actuality powerlifting does not require great power. It requires work, and strength, however, most of the time the lifters move that weight at a slow pace. Usually that is the same case with most individuals at your average gym, there will be some strong people that move heavy amounts of weight, but usually at a slow pace which does not transfer that strength to power. Those strength based exercises performed at slow controlled rates, can reduce athletic performance, because of the recruitment of muscle fibers.

SPEED = Distance Traveled / Per Unit of Time

In most team sports, the determining factors for playing time and distinction is Speed and Power. Those two factors can really separate athletes from good to great or bad to good. Oftentimes, when somebody sees a large individual they will say things like, "You should play football" and if it is a tall person they say, "You should play basketball." Those two sports both require great amounts of speed and power, especially at the offensive and defensive line positions, and at all positions in today's game of basketball.

It is imperative that speed training is a huge staple in any program. Lifting heavy weight is great and all, however, if you cannot move that weight fast, or move your body fast, that big weight is not really doing anything to help with athletic ability.

AGILITY – A sport specific movement, that will require an athlete to have a change of direction that is caused from the sport specific environment.

There are a few different things that can affect an athlete's agility, like the amount of experience or training, their size, muscular fitness, and coordination.
Athletes that possess great agility and quickness levels are often the ones that will catch our eyes during a game, and in practice. They have the ability to stop and then start back at close to the same velocity, or the ability to plant one of their feet at the last second and change direction with great velocity.

COORDINATION – When one is in a stable state, and equal and opposing forces cancel all forces.

Balance is going to require several different systems of the body, including the central nervous system, the peripheral nervous system, visionary components, and vestibular. In sports, our goal is to improve the athletes Dynamic Equilibrium through balance. Dynamic Equilibrium is not necessarily when all net forces equal zero (like Static Equilibrium) but instead it is what will allow the body and nervous system to manage all forces, allowing the athlete to become balanced in the action of a game or practice.

Constructing a Training Program

Offseason Planning

Facility design, layout, and organization

Legality and negligence

Season calendar for strength programs

Sport specific warm ups and stretching (dynamic and static)

Maxing out – what lifts? How many reps?

Understanding the different phases of weight training:

⇒ **Phase 1:** Hypertrophy Phase / General Preparation (high volume, low intensity)

⇒ **Phase 2:** Basic Strength (moderate volume, high intensity)

⇒ **Phase 3:** Strength-Power (low volume, very high intensity)

⇒ **Phase 4:** Peaking / Maintenance

⇒ **Phase 5:** Active Rest (very low volume, very low intensity)

Volume = sets and reps

Intensity = weight and speed / pace

Offseason Planning

- Offseason training starts approx. 2 weeks after the season ends.

- All offseason dates need to be given to the athletes before the last week of regular season -- so they have time to schedule appropriately.

- Below is a list of important dates that should be the focus when planning an offseason strength program.

    - **Training Dates:** MAX days, Athletic testing dates, speed training, 4-5 days a week training, weigh in dates, conditioning test.

    - **Competition Dates:** District or region lift offs.

- **Fundraising Events:** lift-a-thons are a great fundraiser.

- As the strength coach, you should find **professional development** opportunities. This field is growing and new information is crucial in helping the athletes grow, and continue to grow this profession.

Facility Design, Layout, and Organization

- Ceiling height should be at least 12-14 feet high for explosive movements, such as box jumps & other plyometric training.

- Room needs to be in an area with temperature control and ventilation. The goal is to have no higher than 60% humidity to prevent bacterial build ups, and equipment damages.

- Flooring should be a mix of rubber floor and turf if possible (Turf is unrealistic for a lot of programs). This helps with several factors including: cleaning requirements, an athlete's health, and injury prevention (absorbs impact).

- Mirrors should be at least 6 inches from any equipment and 20 inches above the floor.

- All free weight equipment should be placed along the walls of the facility with a minimum 6 inches separating each.

- There should be a minimum clearance of 3 feet between all pieces of equipment in the facility. This allows for traffic flow, safely loading and unloading weights, and enough room to perform the exercises correctly.

- Keep the weight room organized and clean at all times, it allows for better athletic performance and more effect training sessions. (Weights in numerical order, benches inside racks, barbells in a rack or hung up, dumb bells / KB on a rack in order, bands hung up, everything wiped down daily AND AFTER EACH USE.)

Legality and Negligence

- There is always an Assumption of Risk. This is why it is always best to have a qualified / Certified Strength Coach on your staff.

- Athletes must be aware of risks with strength and conditioning activities when they are not performed with proper technique and training.

- It is recommended to sign a statement to provide awareness (usually only in facilities outside of the school building and not school operated), and make sure a parent meeting is held about the structure and all that comes with this program.

- Liability:

  ⇒ Must take steps to prevent injury (strength coach's number one job).

  ⇒ Act accordingly when an injury occurs (follow proper rehab instructions).

- Negligence:

  ⇒ Failure to act with proper standard of care, may lead to injury or damage to an athlete.

- Correct Standard of Care:

  ⇒ The expectation of the strength coach based on their certifications, training or education.

⇒ Athletes may ask about supplements and nutrition.

⇒ It's important to remember that coaches cannot recommend illegal substances.

- As long as they boost athletic performance, abide by the law, and aren't harmful can they be recommended. However, the most recommended supplement that should be referred is FOOD. Supplements will not help enhance the body's performance without proper food intake.

Season Calendar for Strength Programs

Phase 1: 2 weeks of recovery following the conclusion of the season

This period should be used to recover mentally and physically. From the end of the season until the off-season conditioning program begins the following is suggested:

- Do not gain weight.
- Lose excess body fat.
- Participate in recreational exercise (total inactivity not suggested, or your muscle mass will atrophy).

Phase 1 Notes:

Phase 2: 2 weeks after the season ends through spring practice

Organized lifting workouts and supervised running sessions begin during this period. Specific running times and days should be posted.

<u>Maximum fitness levels can be generated by summer camp if</u>:

- Athletes don't gain excess body fat during the first period -- followed by a proper nutrition plan.

- Athletes sustain disciplined work habits throughout the entire off-season, sporadic training will produce submaximal results, you get what you give (Hardest worker in the room, always).

Phase 2 Notes:

Phase 3: Spring Practice. On field practice 4-5 days a week and final phase of program 3 days a week.

At this point the player should be in good running and conditioning shape in order to meet the needs of on field practice work.

- The off-season workout to this point should help prevent non contact and some contact injuries from occurring.
- Final Phase of the program is active rest and maintenance, 3 days a week during spring practice, very low volume and higher weight.

Phase 3 Notes:

Phase 4: End of spring. 1 week off for recovery. Start of summer condition, in preparation for the season, and continue into the season.

8 weeks of summer training plus 10 weeks of regular season, plus a potential playoff push.

- It is during this period that a player needs to be strongest and most fit. This is the most important period to emphasize strength and conditioning.

- Maximum strength and conditioning levels can be attained and maintained if:

⇒ Players remain disciplined on and off the field.

⇒ Sound nutritional habits and adequate rest are crucial.

⇒ Players give maximum effort each and every training session.

⇒ Practice fast and play fast to develop fitness levels needed to play the game.

Phase 4 Notes:

Sport Specific Warm-Ups and Stretching (Dynamic and Static)

Dynamic Stretching:

√ This type of stretching is best used for pre-competition
√ Involves Speed, Agility, Plyometric

Benefits before competition include:

- Warms body up
- Prepares muscles for contraction and relaxation
- Increases heart rate
- Loosens joints to allow for full range of motion

Static Stretching:

√ This type of stretching is best used in post-competition
√ This includes stretching and holding a specific muscle
√ Usually, 10-30 seconds
√ No ballistic movements

Benefits for this include:

- Increases overall flexibility
- Reduces recovery time for muscles
- Injury prevention

Sport Specific Warm-Up:

Should relate to game situations, and sport skills used. Benefits for sport specific warm-ups:

- Improved speed
- More power output
- Better coordination
- Overall better sports performance
- Injury Prevention

Maxing Out – What lifts? How many reps?:

- Bench - 2-3 reps (use conversion sheet to find 1rm)
- Squat - 2-3 reps (use conversion sheet to find 1rm)
- Power Clean - 1 rep
- Deadlift - 1 rep

These are the core lifts to max out to start and retest throughout your program.

They are fundamental in power and strength, they also have the most football related output.

Understanding the Different Phases of Weight Training

Phase 1: Hypertrophy Phase / General Preparation (high volume, low intensity)

- Geared towards reconditioning the body, increasing lean body mass, and increasing muscular endurance.

- Reps in this phase are in the 8-15 range, for 3-4 sets, with the weight being lighter.

- The percentage of the athletes max out should range from 55%-70% on the core lifts (Squat, Power Clean, Deadlift, and Bench Press).

- In some cases, the percentage layout will not be applicable. For example, throughout the program powerclean will always have some sets which will be completed at 90%-95% regardless of the phase.

- The aim in this phase is to teach (or re-teach) different movements, especially those which will be the foundation of your lifting program (Squat, Power Clean, Deadlift, and Bench Press), as well as to make sure the athletes recover from the season, and are able to recover from any injuries that may have taken place.

Phase 2: Basic Strength (moderate volume, high intensity)

- The goal here is to increase specific strength for the athletes as the foundation for future power / high intensity work.
- The reps and sets for this phase are generally in 3-5 sets of 5-8 reps.
- The percentage of the athletes max out should range from 70%-80% on the core lifts (Squat, Power Clean, Deadlift, and Bench Press).

Phase 3: Strength-Power (low volume, very high intensity)

- The athlete trains using 3-5 sets of 2-5 reps in the main lifts of their program. Auxiliary lifts will have a higher volume and intensity still.
- The Percentage of the athletes max out should range from 80%-95% on the core lifts (Squat, Power Clean, Deadlift, and Bench Press).
- In this phase, generally due to the increased strength the athlete has experienced but also the decreased fatigue because of the lower volume, the athlete can display greater power.

Phase 4: Peaking / Maintenance

- Train using 1-3 sets of 1-3 reps, with high intensity.
- The key here is to not wear out the athletes and allow them to regain full stamina before they compete (spring practice).

Phase 5: Active Rest (very low volume, very low intensity)

- Take a week off of heavy duty lifting.
- Play recreational sports and games to keep endurance levels up and prevent atrophy.

There will be NO GUARANTEES

When it comes to getting bigger, stronger, faster, and creating a great strength and conditioning program, it is all about the amount of work the athletes and coaches are willing to put into it. There is no magic formula, other than working hard, and smart about the approach to it.

There is no one "right way" or no one "wrong way" to do it. There are a lot of great strength coaches in the world and we almost always have a different way to approach it, just like different head coaches have different approaches to their operations. A couple things to caution on is to approach this with science, expert advice (not just anyone can be an EFFECTIVE strength coach, find someone with formal training or education in the field), and the athletes best interest in mind.

When keeping the athletes best interest in mind it is important to remember that we are trying to:

1. Prevent future injuries of athletes.

2. Develop athletes so coaches can put the best possible product on the court or field.

3. Create a great culture of competition, teamwork, and winning.

4. Remember that this is not a "More is better" area. Use the science we have available and do what is necessary. We do

not need to punish athletes with more physical work, or see how sore we can make them. That is an old school way, and is not necessarily the best way to approach strength and conditioning.

Coaching Tips:

- Every athlete's body is different. It is important to remember that they will all develop at different times and to factor in different key factors like their diet and starting BMI.

- Stay positive and continue to encourage your athletes when some athletes don't demonstrate results as fast as others.

Importance of a Spotter

When it comes to establishing a Strength & Conditioning program it is important to have a spotter that matches the ability of the athlete they are spotting. For example, if a player benches 250 pounds it is important to have a spotter that can lift the weight if necessary.

A spotter is teammate, coach, or trainer that is aware of safety procedures and proper technique. This person's first job is to make sure that reps are completed safely, and with good technique. Each lift will usually have very specific actions the spotter must take in order to help the lifting athlete.

Coaching Tip: Never let a player lift alone

Before performing any lift, athletes should **ALWAYS** have a spotter, in the case of failure. The failure to have a spotter, and spotter performing their job correctly can lead to serious injury.

Every spotter needs to be trained in the correct procedures to follow for each station. Never assume they know what they are doing until they are trained.

Breathing is Vital

Breathing correctly during a lift, especially heavy lifting, is necessary to make sure the blood is being oxygenated while circulating to specific working muscles -- so waste products are removed and the effort is rewarded with maximum results.

If an athlete holds their breath during an exercise, they can increase their blood pressure to dangerous levels which can result in an injury. It is important for a spotter to watch for proper breathing techniques while lifting and help remind them to breathe.

If the person lifting realizes they are not breathing correctly or feeling light headed then they need to stop immediately and adjust the weights.

Inhale on the release. Exhale on the lift.

Reflection Notes:

Reflection Notes – Continued:

Reflection Notes – Continued:

Reflection Notes – Continued:

Chapter 2:
Daily Mobility

Daily Mobility is something that should not be taken for granted. Improving your Mobility is completing different than lifting weights, so it is important to remember that it will take time to improve and maintain. Your joints were designed to move a certain way so never force it. Make sure your players know to always listen to their body

Coaching Tip: Stay active no matter how old you get.

Incorporate daily mobility exercises to any workout. It does not need to be long but it is a vital component to include something. When coaching and training athletes it is important to remember to develop them as a whole athlete not isolate their potential.

Recommendation: Yoga is a very effective component to incorporate into any workout regimen.

Dynamic Mobility

This is something that has really become a huge trend in the last 30 years with a lot of sports teams. Dynamics stretches are movements that prepare your muscles, ligaments to get you ready to move around. A good dynamic warm up is anywhere from 5 to 15 minutes long and the intensity is low to moderate range.

Dynamic Stretching:

- ★ This type of stretching is best used for pre-competition
- ★ Involves Speed, Agility, Plyometric
- ★ Benefits before competition include:
    - Warms body up
    - Prepares muscles for contraction and relaxation
    - Increases heart rate
    - Loosens joints to allow for full range of motion

Static Mobility

Static stretches were the "norm" for starting practices years ago. Coaches would instruct players to do them before and after practice. Research shows that static mobility may possibly decrease your athlete's performance by decreasing the ability of a muscule to produce force. Doing these at the wrong time could result in a serious sport injury.

However, Static Stretches are great to incorporate during a cool down period or creating it as part of a normal routine at the end of each practice, which might help prevent injury.

Static Stretching:

- This type of stretching is best used in post-competition
- This includes stretching and holding a specific muscle
- Hold a stretch for approximately 10-30 seconds
- No ballistic movements
- Benefits for this include:
  - Increases overall flexibility
  - Reduces recovery time for muscles
  - Injury prevention

Flexibility

Flexibility has stood the test of time in the Strength and Conditioning realm and is still going strong today. This is all about the (ROM) Range of Motion. This helps get your muscles ready to stretch. Muscles are like rubber bands, if you over stretch them or push them to the limits they will tear, snap, or break. How to prevent muscle injuries: proper stretching and maintaining good form.

Proper Stretching = Improved Flexibility

You have to remember to stretch until you have a comfortable stretch not over do it to the point of pain.

Not sure if you want to talk about the 3 different types of flexibility.

Injury Prevention

Injury Prevention is a way to try to reduce or prevent the severity of an injury before it occurs.

This is a topic that always comes up more and more with sports today. Twenty to thirty years ago basketball teams weren't playing five to seven games during a weekend and baseball teams didn't play seven baseball games in five days. People ask why there are so many injuries in sports today compared to previous years, it is because we are pushing athletes to the brink of not walking away from a sport after their high school career is over.

There are many different ways to help with injury prevention – the following are just a few ways and are in no certain order:

- ★ Allow a player to take time off to rest
- ★ Let players take a break during a game "Don't run the wheels off the car"
- ★ Make sure to increase their flexibility
- ★ Strengthen their muscles
- ★ Make sure players use proper techniques while moving
- ★ Make sure players wear the correct gear
- ★ Make sure players don't play through pain -- It does not make them "tougher"

NOTE: The above list is just a recommendation and does not guarantee an injury will not occur. Good Luck!

Reflection Notes:

Reflection Notes – Continued:

Reflection Notes – Continued:

Reflection Notes – Continued:

Chapter 3:
Basic Strength Testing Procedures & Techniques

As a coach, it is important to gage what your players are capable of before implementing a strength and conditioning program. It provides you with a clear starting point that allows you to create a specific program that can be unique to that player. It provides you and the player with a way to document and track improvement, see if they plateau, or see if something isn't working and make adjustments accordingly. There are a few keys attributes that make any regiment successful:

- Accountability
- Focus
- Determination
- Realistic Goals
- Tracking

Accountability + Realistic Goals = Motivation

Accountability is one way to keep players on track. That is why it is important to keep players focused because it will motivate them when they see how much they grow over a certain amount of time. What better way to motivate a player then to let them visually see how they crush their goals?

Bench

Purpose:
The bench press is used as an overall test of upper body strength, including the hips, core, pectoralis major, pectoralis minor, triceps, and deltoids. For example, Football players will be competing one on one with other players and will be required to use both arms to press off a blocker or defender with explosive movement from the upper body.

Applies to the following Sport(s):
Various. Bench Press will be useful to athletes that participate in sports with explosive movements, and use of the upper body.

Applies to the following Position(s):
Various.

Equipment:
- Olympic sized barbell
- Bench, rack or cage
- Safety locks for both sides of the bar
- Enough weight in varied sizes to supply and accommodate the strongest athlete

Spotter:

Before performing any lift, athletes should **ALWAYS** have a spotter, in the case of failure. The failure to have a spotter, and spotter performing their job correctly can lead to serious injury.

- Spotter is standing attentively behind the bar, and above the athlete performing the bench.
- The Spotter should have one hand placed under the bar, and the opposite hand placed over the bar.
- Spotters hand should move in symmetry with the bar, without touching it unless the athlete is unable to successfully lift the weight.
- In that case, wrap both hands around the bar, lift up, and guide the weight onto the rack ensuring it is secure.

Technique:

- Athletes should be lying supine (back on bench).
- Shoulders and hips should have contact with the bench, slight arch in the spine.
- Feet should be firmly against the floor, pressing down (Tell athletes to push their feet through the floor.)
- Hands need to be spaced evenly on the bar (Place end of thumb against the start of the knurl, spread the hand out, close fist, this should give a shoulder or slightly wider than shoulder grip).
- With control, the athlete should lower the bar to their chest, at the nipple line.
- Forcefully push the weight until their arms are fully extended.

Max Out Procedure:

- Athletes should perform a warmup of 5-10 reps with a light load.
- The athlete should perform 2-3 more warm up sets of 3-5 reps with a moderate load.
- Athletes should have a spotter and coach (recorder) present before performing a max out attempt.
- Athlete then performs the attempt, and the coach will decide if the attempt will be recorded based on technique.
- This should be a Hyped-up environment, it is a chance for the players to compete, learn to celebrate with teammates, and win the day!

Alternated Lifts / Modification:

- Dumbbell bench press
- Alternate DB Bench Press
- Push-Ups (Incline, decline, standard)
- Banded Press

Before lifting make sure feet, hips and shoulders are FIRMLY in contact with the surface. Make sure elbows are at a 45-degree angle, and the bar is touching at or just below the nipple line. Both of these will help to better protect the shoulders from injury, and target the pecs more.

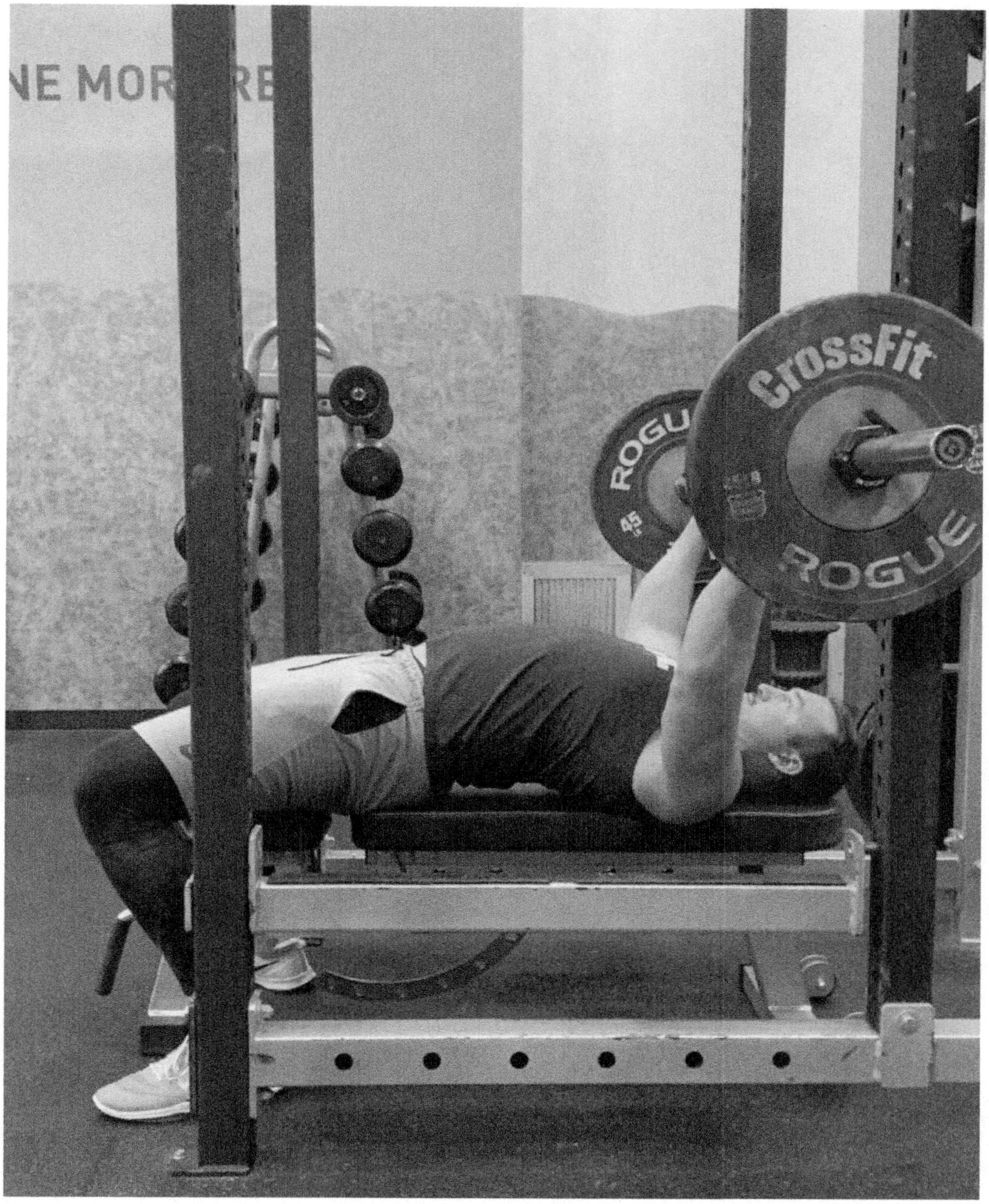

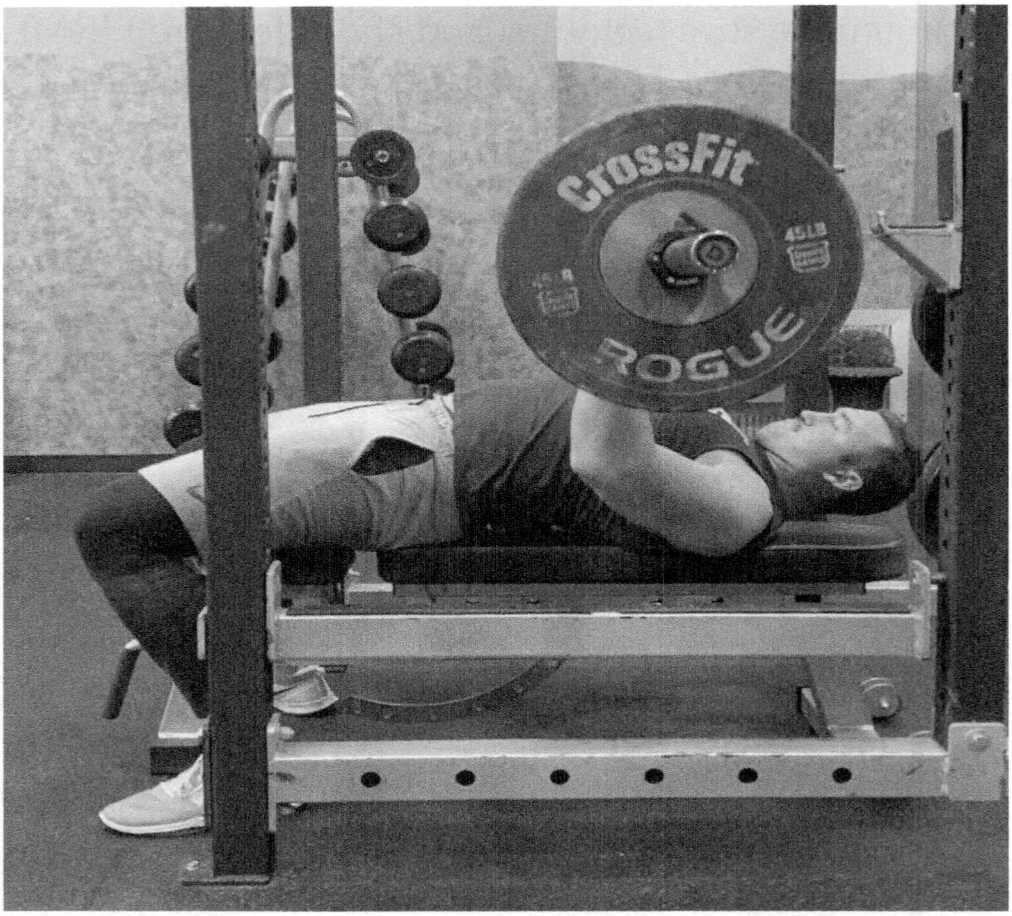
CrossFit
45LB
ROGUE

On the eccentric movement (Downward), the glutes, shoulders and feet, are all in solid contact with the correct surface.

Again, elbows bent at a 45-degree angle, bar at or below the nipple and all points of contact are in place.

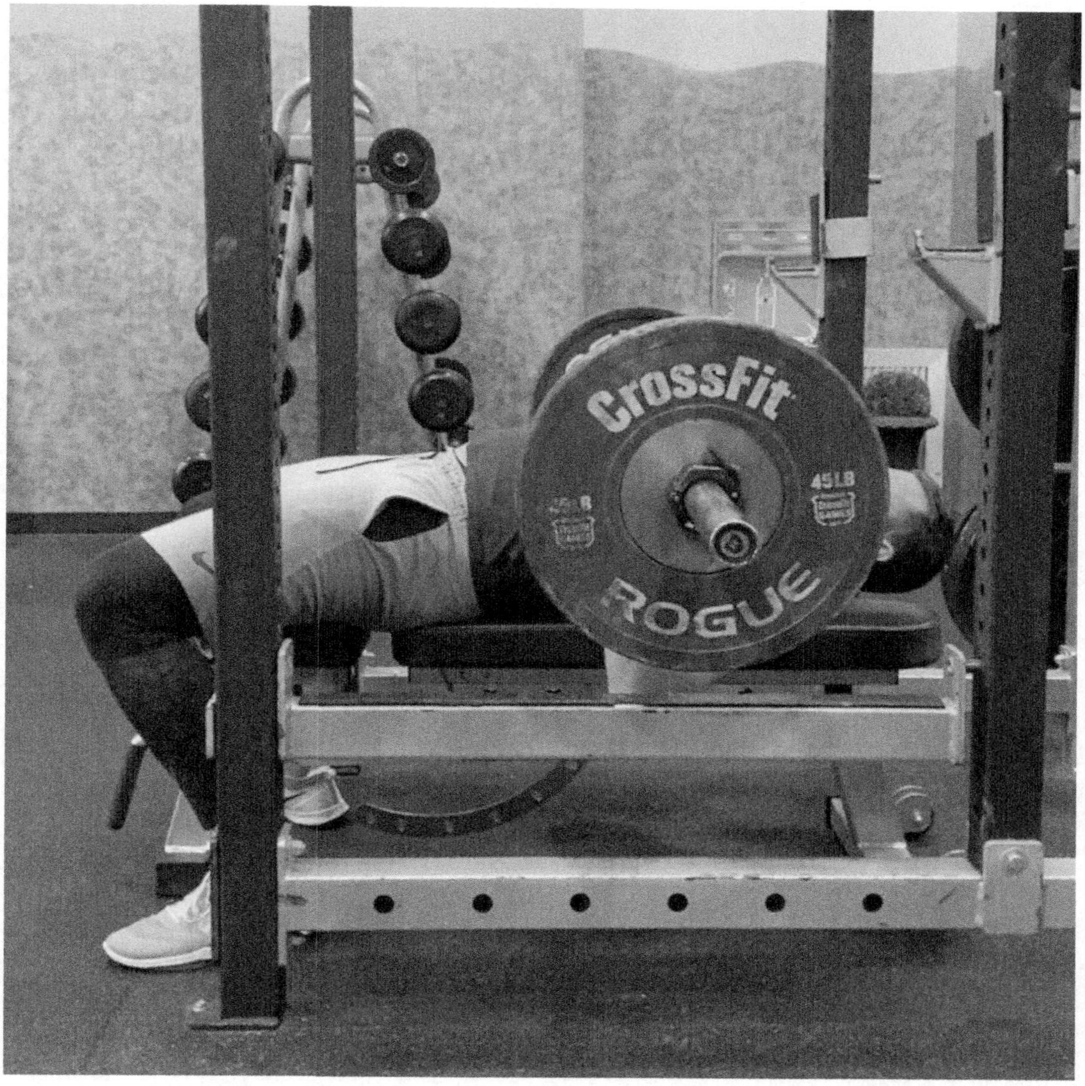

On the drive up, push through the feet and hips. The glutes will have a thrusting movement (Athletes move through their hips in sport, so lift like they play).

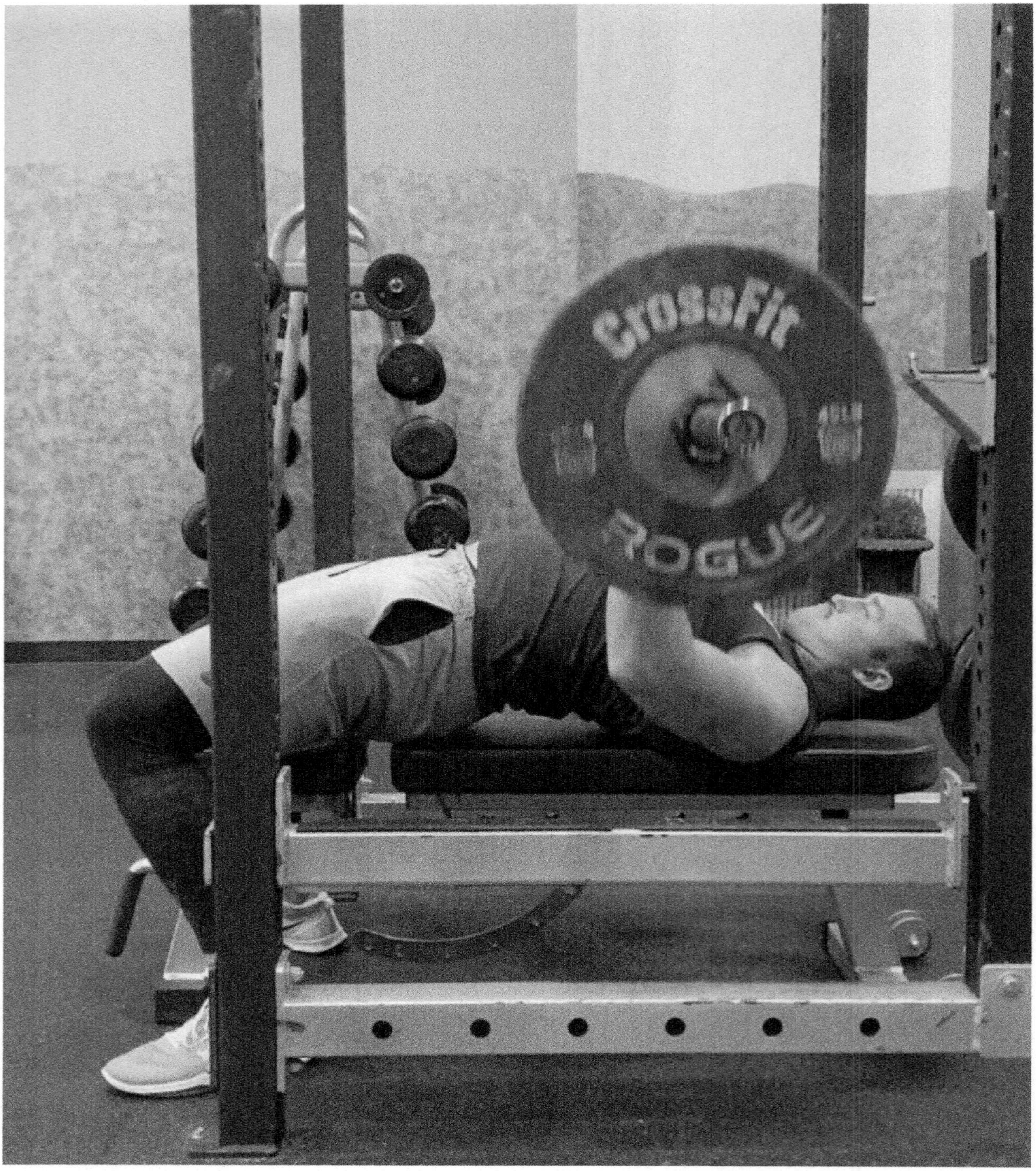

Power/ Hang Clean

Purpose:
The Power and Hang clean is the ultimate weight room test to measure the power and explosiveness of an athlete. These lifts are a multi-joint lift, and use the complete body to perform it correctly. This lift will require many hours of practice in order to master the technique well enough to perform a max out test. It is important to break down all parts of a power clean and so they all individually become the staple of the season and off-season Training Program. These parts include: Deadlift, Power Pull, Hang Pull, and Front Squats.

Applies to the following Sport(s):
Various. Any sport that requires power output from an athlete will benefit abundantly from incorporating the correct use of Power and Hang Cleans.

Applies to the following Position(s):
Various.

Equipment:
- Olympic barbell with revolving sleeves
- Weighted bumper plates of various sizes
- An area with enough open space to perform the lift safely
- Enough weight in varied sizes to supply and accommodate the strongest athlete

Spotter:
There is no great way to spot Power Lifts. The best thing to do, is to be in the general vicinity while being attentive to your teammate performing the lift. That way, if something happens and they need your help or attention you can respond effectively.

Technique:

- In the Power Clean, the athlete will start from the floor in a deadlift position (chest and head up, butt down, bar against shin).
- For the Hang Clean, the athlete will start in a standing position holding the bar, bringing the bar down to above the knee brushing against the thigh while keeping the head and chest up, and pushing the hips and butt back.
- At this point, in both variations the athlete is going to perform ONE fluid motion from the floor or above the knee to the catch position (bottom of Front squat).
- Rise from the squat.
- The athlete will reset the lift from the starting point.

Max Out Procedure:

- Athletes should perform a warmup of 5-10 reps with a light load.
- The Athlete should perform 2-3 more warmup sets of 3-5 reps with a moderate load.
- Athletes should have a spotter and coach (recorder) present before performing max out attempt.
- Athlete then performs the attempt, and the coach will decide if the attempt will be recorded based on technique.
- This should be a Hyped-Up environment, it is a chance for the players to compete, learn to celebrate with teammates, and win the day!

Alternated Lifts / Modification:

- PVC Pipe
- Broom Sticks
- Kettle Bells
- Dumb Bells

Coaching Points:

- Remember this lift is broken down into multiple parts. Perfect each one, and put it together.
- If you notice your athlete struggling with a particular movement, they should add an extra emphasis on that part.

Power Clean Breakdown:

- Hip Swings
- Upright Rows
- High Pull

POWER CLEAN START

Start in a deadlift position. The Hips are back, bar is against legs, head in an upward position, and spine is neutral.

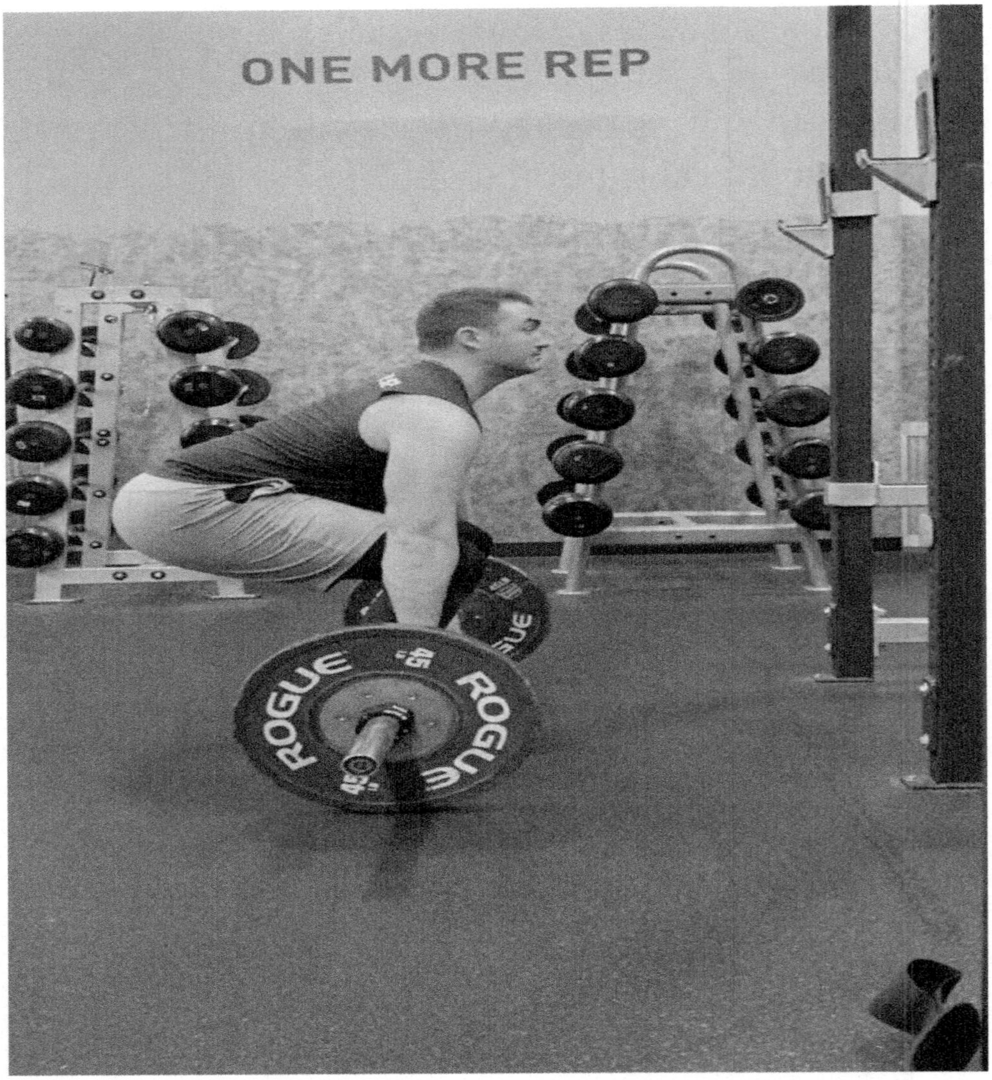

HANG CLEAN START

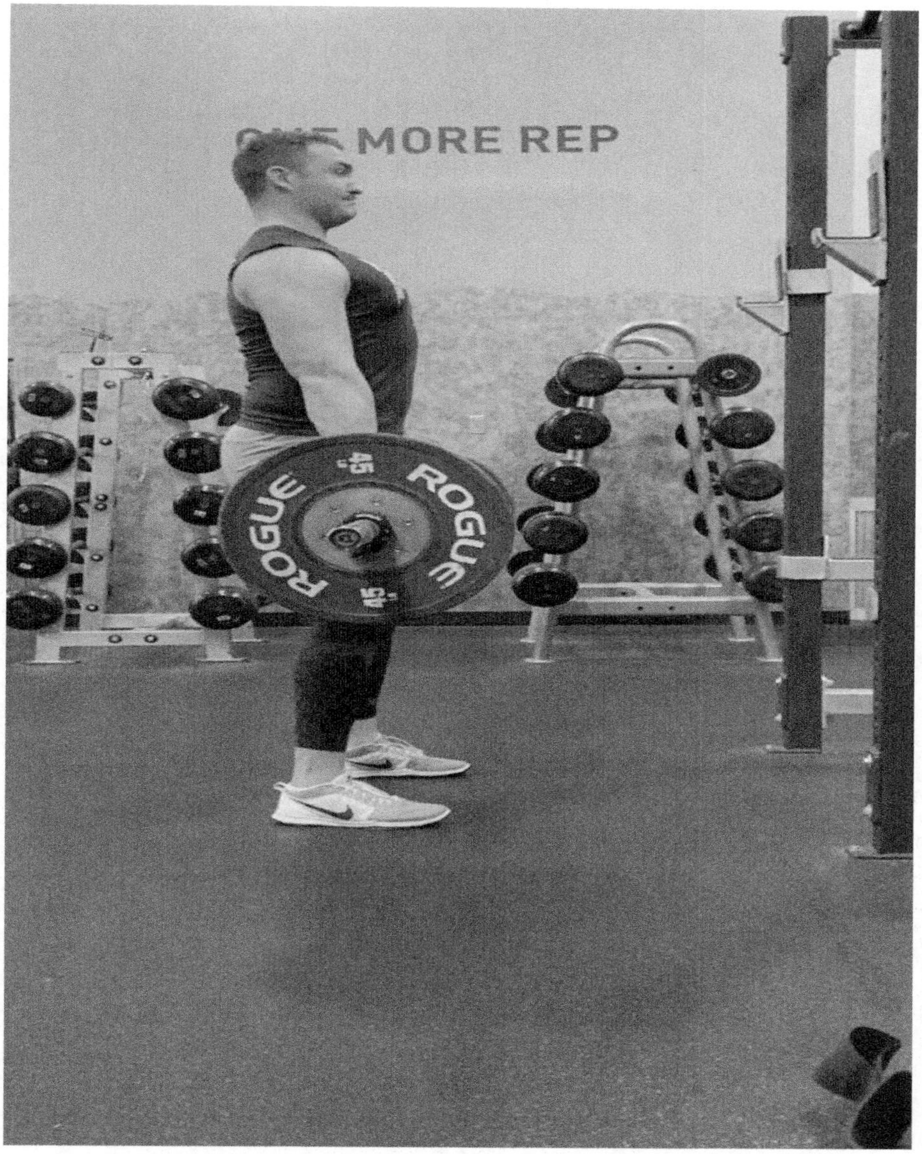

As the athlete drives up, keep the bar against the body, the spine in a neutral position, and one fluid motion.

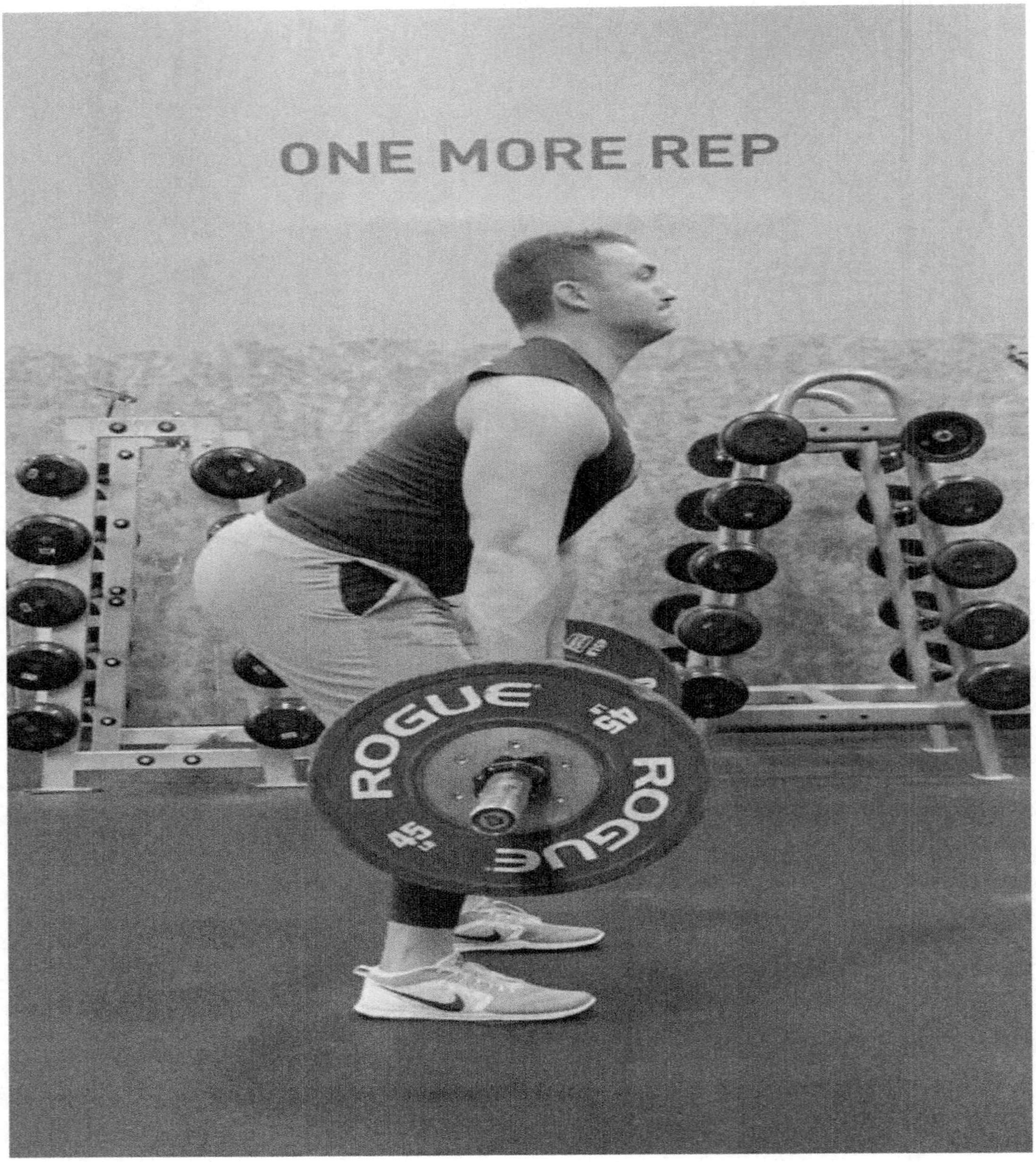

The athlete should drive up through the feet, shrugging the bar up with maximum force.

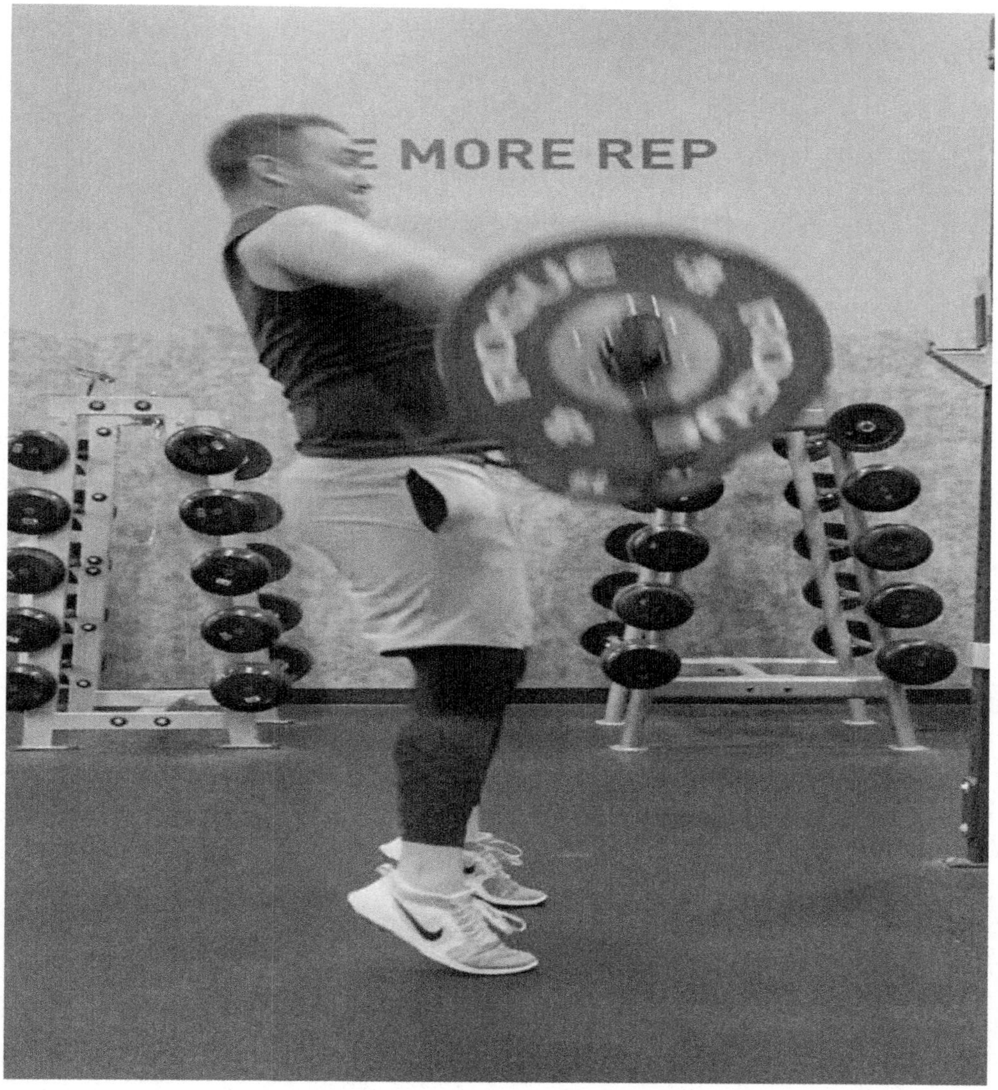

In the fluid motion, the elbows will rise up, keeping the bar on an even plain. This is the last part before the snatch and catch.

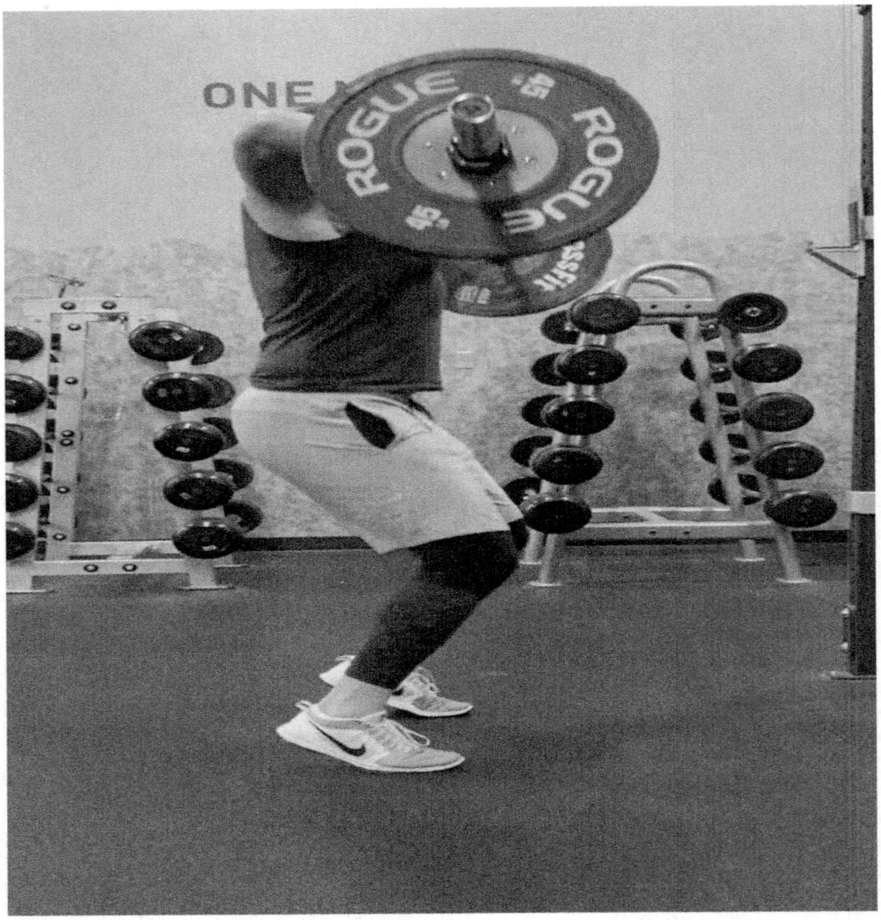

The Catch Position -- With good hip mobility, and body movement the catch should happen in the same position as the hole of a front squat.

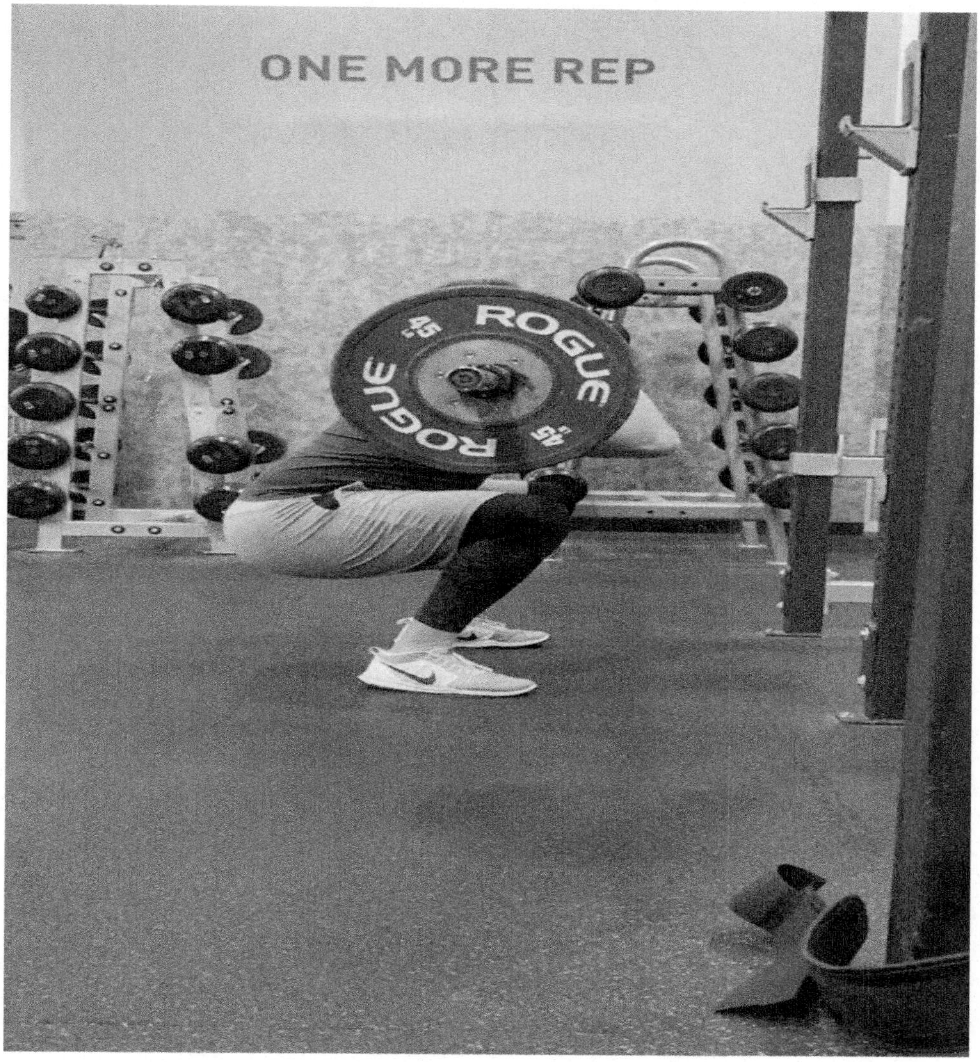

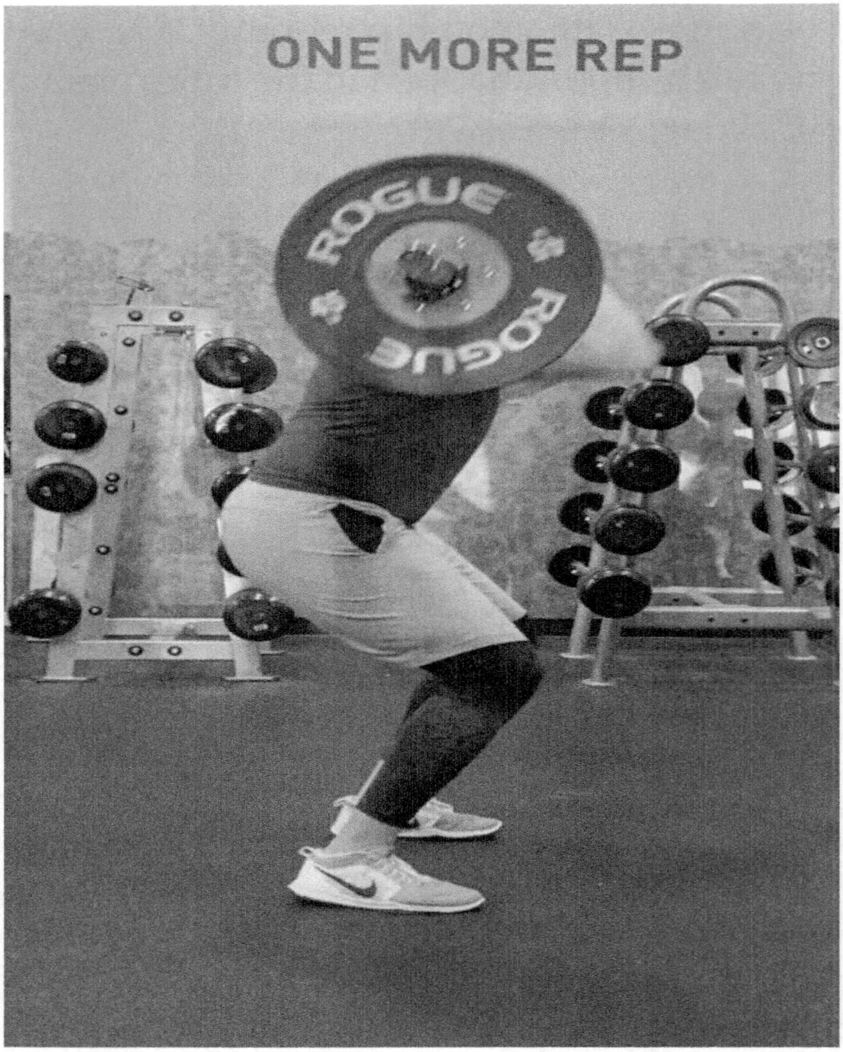
ONE MORE REP
ROGUE
ROGUE

Back / Front Squat

Purpose:
The Squat is a true test of how strong the athletes lower body and core really is. When squatting, the athlete is controlling a tremendous amount of weight from the top of their torso, all the way down to their feet. When an athlete can start to squat a heavy load, through a full range of motion, it has the possibility to translate to incredible athletic feats that can include things like increased speed, a higher vertical jump, and more explosive movements.

Applies to the following Sport(s):
All Sports. All athletes can benefit from squatting, when performed correctly.

Applies to the following Position(s):
All Positions and athletes.

Equipment:
- Olympic sized Barbell
- Enough weight in varied sizes to supply and accommodate the strongest athlete
- Two safety clips for both ends of the bar
- A strong, sturdy rack or cage with adjustable bar racks and spotter racks
- A flat surface for the athlete to stand and perform lift

Spotter:
When spotting a teammate on the squat, be prepared to be up close and personal, as social distancing is not possible. When an athlete is going to spot a teammate on the squat, they will stand directly behind the athlete performing the lift, with their hands under the lifters arms, supporting their chest (Hands should be placed on the upper portion of the chest, near the shoulders). This is to keep the lifter's spine in a neutral position, and keep it from dropping which can cause serious injury. (If the spotter starts to feel the lifter fall forward, or start to drop their back forward, they should pull in an upward motion on the lifter's chest/shoulder area.) As the lifter goes through a full range of motion, so does the spotter, as they will mirror the movement of the lifter. When the reps and set are complete, the spotter will grab the bar and guide the lifter into the rack until the bar is secure.

Technique:

- Athletes will walk into the Rack towards the bar, and place hands about 6 inches outside of shoulders.
- With Hands spaced evenly apart, the athlete will slide under the bar and place it on top of the rear deltoid, below the neck.
- The athlete will then pick up the bar, take 1-2 steps back and place feet just out of the hips, with feet at a 45-degree angle.
- With a spotter present, the Athlete will start to descend.
- The first motion should be to push the hips back. With that motion, the knees will start to bend with involuntary movement.
- Remember to make sure the athlete is keeping their head up (pick a spot on the wall and stare at it).
- Big Chest.
- Big Butt.

Max Out Procedure:

- Athletes should perform a warmup of 5-10 reps with a light load.
- The Athlete should perform 2-3 more warm up sets of 3-5 reps with a moderate load.
- Athletes should have a spotter and coach (recorder) present before performing max out attempt.
- Athlete then performs the attempt, and the coach will decide if the attempt will be recorded based on technique.
- This should be a Hyped-Up environment, it is a chance for the players to compete, learn to celebrate with teammates, and win the day!

Alternated Lifts / Modification:

- Goblet Squats (Dumbbell, Kettlebell)
- Body Squats
- Pistol Squats
- Single Leg Squats
- Split squat

To start, make sure feet are under the hips, toes slightly out, firm grip on the bar, and feet are aligned with one another.
The first movement should be a hip hinge. The hips should start to push back while keeping the chest as big as possible while staring straight ahead or slightly up. The weight should be in the heels.

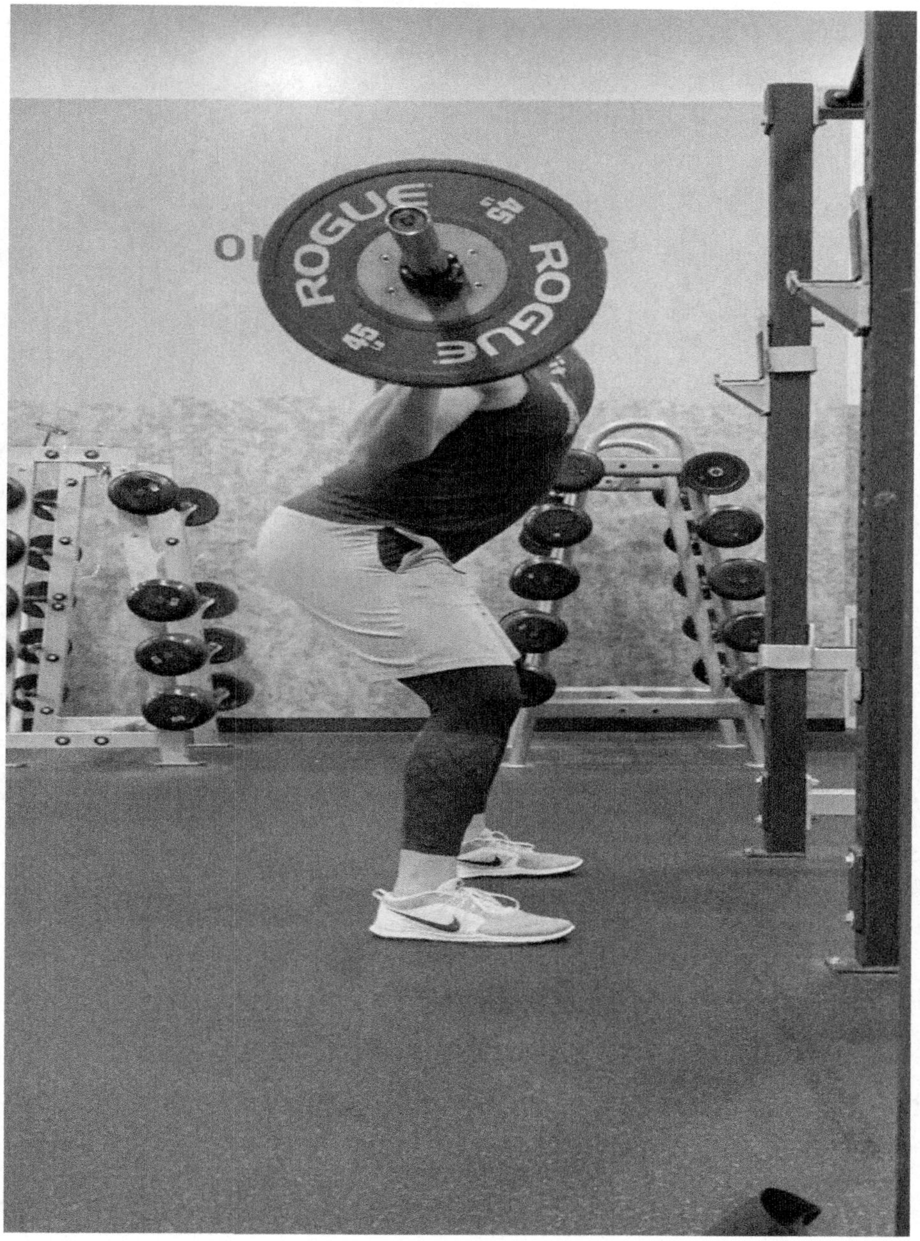

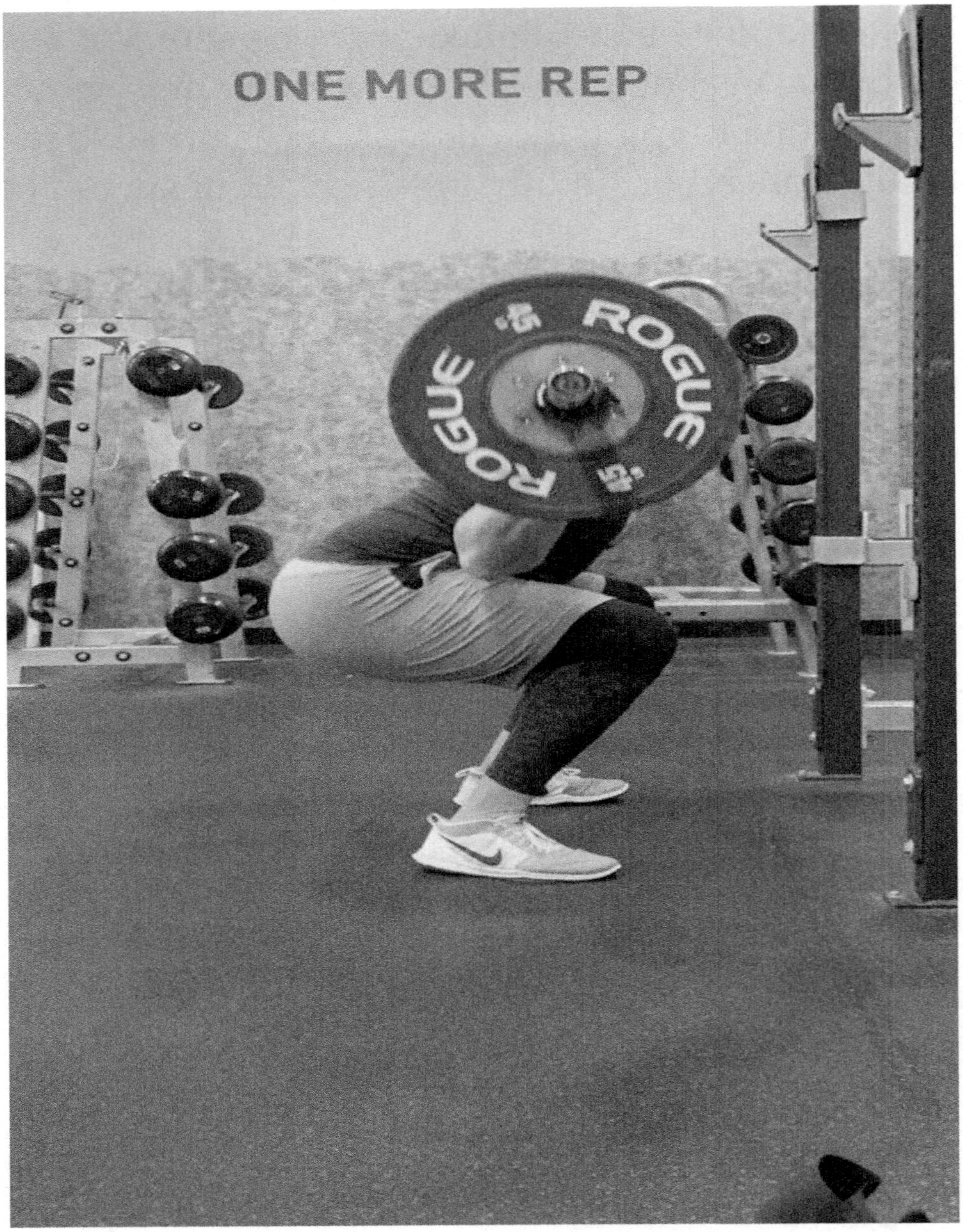

The “hole” or bottom of the lift should finish with the knees behind or right above the toes, the spine in a neutral position, and as close to or below parallel. This will vary by player, as each body is different anatomically.

For a Front Squat, make sure the weight is resting on the shoulders, not the hands. The elbows should be straight out, and parallel to the ground.

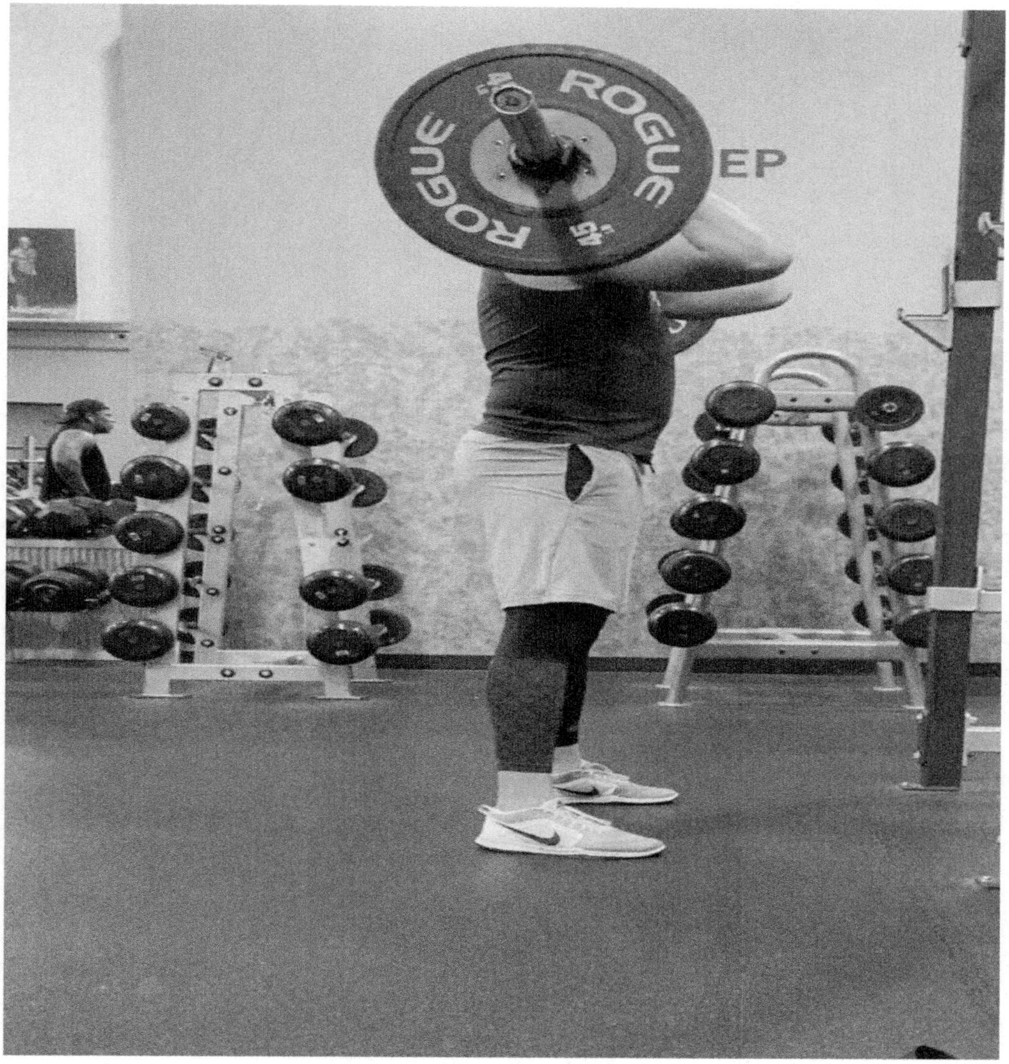

The elbows should stay up and the hip hinge is the same as back squat as is the weight being transferred to the heels of the athlete.

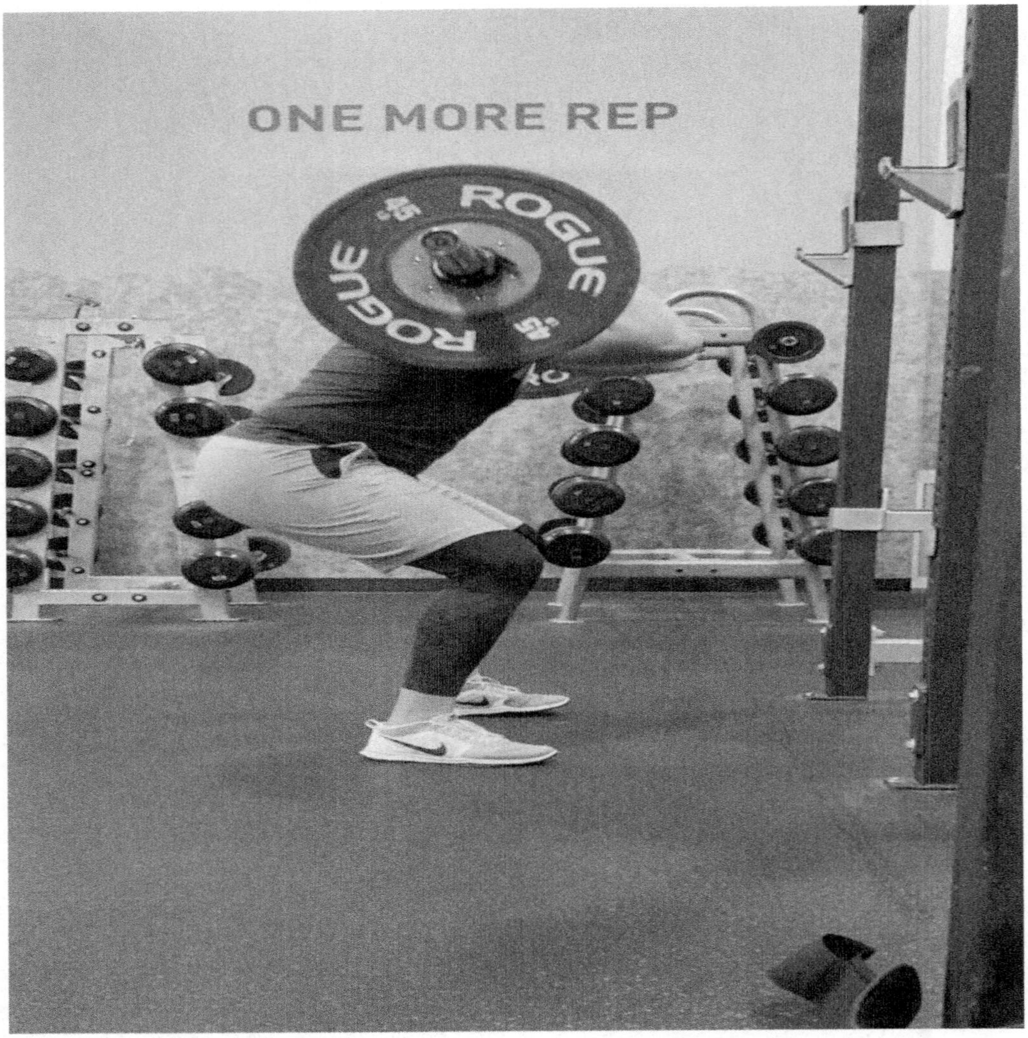

The bottom of the lift, ebows still in the correct position, weight in the heels, and the spine is neutral.

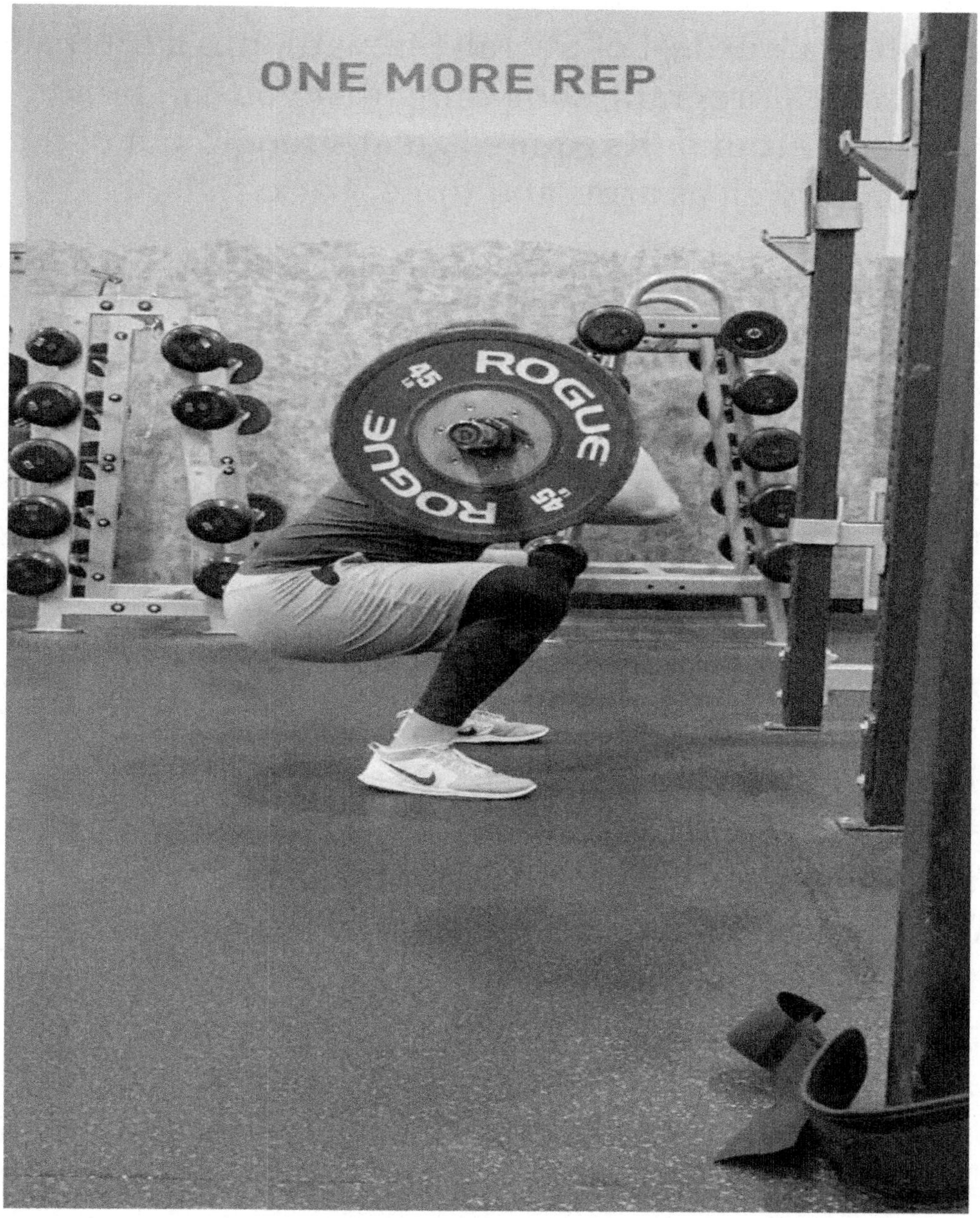

DeadLift

Purpose:
The Deadlift is a true test of overall Strength. It is a lift that can be a centerpiece of a program, something that you can build everything else around. It requires great strength out of the legs, core, lumbar, as well as arms and upper back.

Applies to the following Sport(s):
Various. All athletes will benefit from deadlifting, properly, throughout a strength program.

Applies to the following Position(s):
Various. All athletes will benefit from deadlifting, properly, throughout a strength program.

Equipment:
- Olympic sized Barbell
- Enough weight in varied sizes to supply and accommodate the strongest athlete
- Two safety clips for both ends of the bar
- A flat surface for the athlete to stand and perform lift

Spotter:
When Spotting the deadlift, the spotter will need to stand behind the athlete performing the lift. The spotter will take their far hand and place it on the lower back of the athlete just above the glutes, and the spotters near hand will go under the athlete's arm placed center on their chest. When the spotter gets into the correct position, they can now push down on the lower back, and pull with their near hand on the chest. This position allows for the spotter to assist in making sure the bottom half of the lifter does not rise too quickly while dropping their chest and head causing improper form and possible injury to the lower back.

Technique:

- The athlete needs to have their feet under or just outside of their hips.
- The athlete will place their hands just outside of their hips (feet if a little wide in stance).
- The most important ques for the Athlete to follow will be to keep their chest and head up, butt down, and the bar against their shin.
- The Athlete needs to drive through their legs first.
- Once the bar is lifted off the ground and around the pelvic area, the athlete wants to drive the hips forward, while retracting their scapulas (this is where a lot of the important benefits from deadlift come in).
- The athlete should control the weight and bar back down to the floor, as putting it down is also part of the lift.

Max Out Procedure:

- Athletes should perform a warmup of 5-10 reps with a light load.
- The Athlete should perform 2-3 more warm up sets of 3-5 reps with a moderate load.
- Athletes should have a spotter and coach (recorder) present before performing max out attempt.
- Athlete then performs the attempt, and the coach will decide if the attempt will be recorded based on technique.
- This should be a Hyped-Up environment, it is a chance for the players to compete, learn to celebrate with teammates, and win the day!

Alternated Lifts / Modification:

- Dumbbell / Kettlebell Deadlift
- Banded Deadlifts (Place a resistance band under feet, and use that instead of a bar).

The Hips are back, bar is against legs, head in an upward position and spine is neutral.

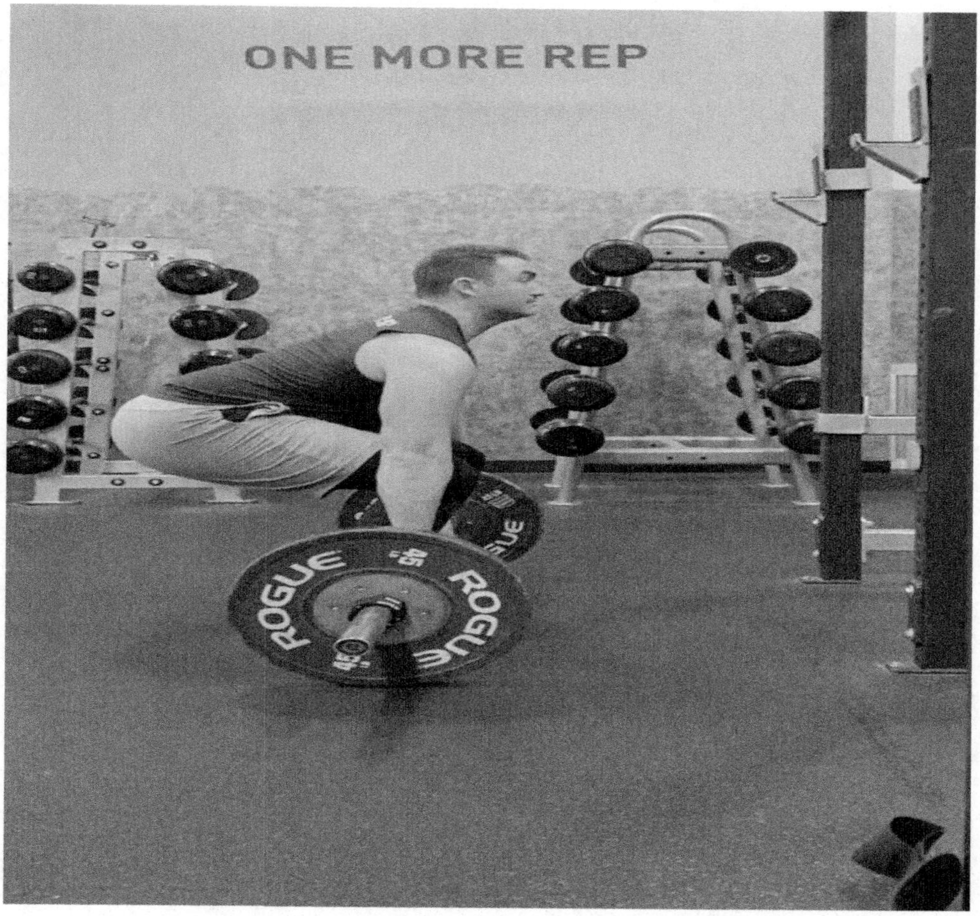

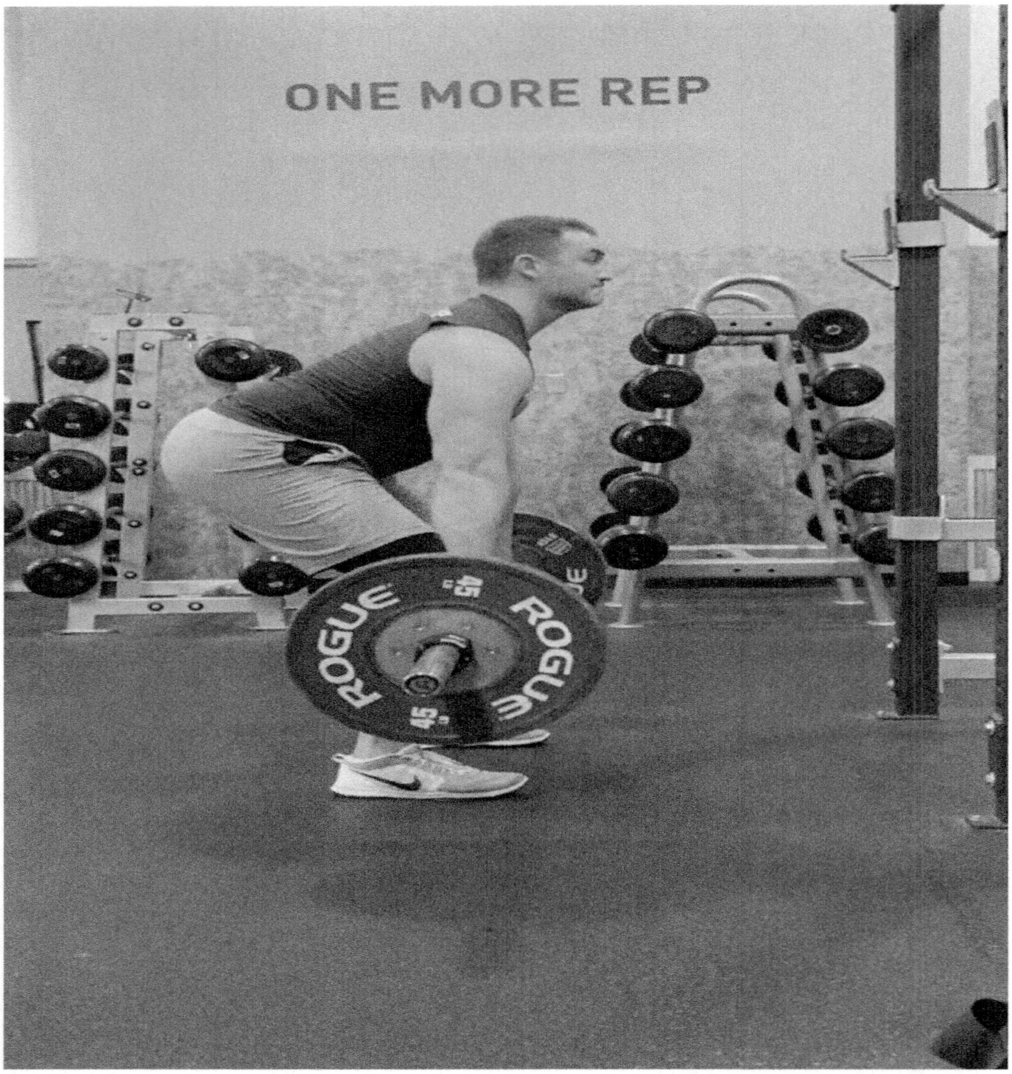
ONE MORE REP
ROGUE
ROGUE
45

The top of the lift should be the shoulders rotated back, and the hips pushed forward. Putting the weight down is half the lift, so do not drop from the top.

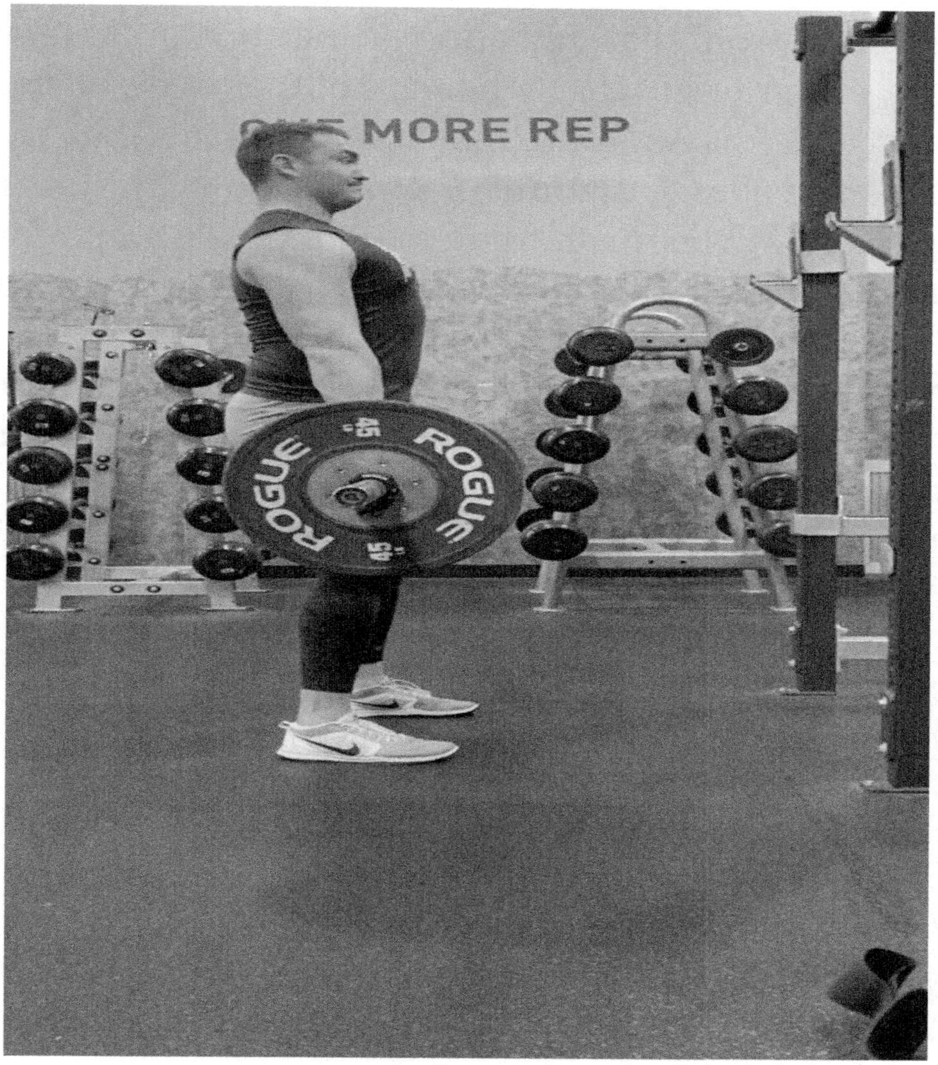

Barbell / Standard Hip Thruster

Purpose:
Every coach should understand that the power an athlete produces comes from their hips (including core, and glutes). It is the athletes center of gravity, where all of their weight should be held evenly. This is even more relevant to athletes that are required to have a large amount of power and explosion, like football players. When developing a football player, strength coaches are looking to develop whole body athletes with huge emphasis on certain areas of their bodies. Strength Coaches should be trying to develop the areas which create the most explosive athletes: Quadriceps, Hamstrings, Gluteus Maximus (Butt), and Core. The Hip Thruster is a must have for development of all of those listed above. It puts a real emphasis on the Glutes and Hamstring, while providing a great core exercise. It also will help develop hip mobility, which can aid in decreased injuries and increased power.

Applies to the following Sport(s):
Various. Most sports require lower body and core strength.

Applies to the following Position(s):
Various. More specifically, every player on a football team should routinely perform Hip Thrusters.

Equipment:

- Bench
- Olympic Barbell
- Enough weight in varied sizes to supply and accommodate the strongest athlete
- Two safety clips for both ends of the bar
- A flat surface for the athlete to perform lift
- It helps to have a towel or pad to place on the bar

Spotter:

No spotter required. It is always advised to have a teammate watching, in the case of an emergency.

Technique:

- The athlete will need to set a sturdy bench horizontal to the barbell.
- The athlete will sit on the floor in front of the bench with the bar in front of their feet.
- The Athlete will need to roll the bar up their legs and over their pelvis area.
- The Bar should be sitting on the waistline.
- It can be helpful to wrap a towel or pad around the bar, this will help the athletes comfort.
- Once the bar is at the waistline, the athlete will need to bring their feet into their body and place them firmly on the ground.
- Once their feet are set, the scapulas should be the only part of the body in contact with the bench.
- With two hands placed on the bar, feet and scapulas in place the athlete will press their pelvis towards the air, squeezing their glutes at the top.

- After each glute squeeze at the top of the lift, the athlete will control the weight back down. Once the Butt touches the ground, it should immediately explode back up for another rep, until the set is complete.

Max Out Procedure:
There is no Max Out for this lift. This is a lift that should be incorporated with push days, or lower body days as often as possible.

Alternated Lifts / Modification:
- Single leg glute bridge
- Regular glute bridge (no weight)
- Banded glute bridge
- Dumbbell Hip Thruster

The scapulas should be in contact with the bench, the feet should be pressed FIRMLY against the ground, and the bar is sitting on the pelvis area at the waist line.

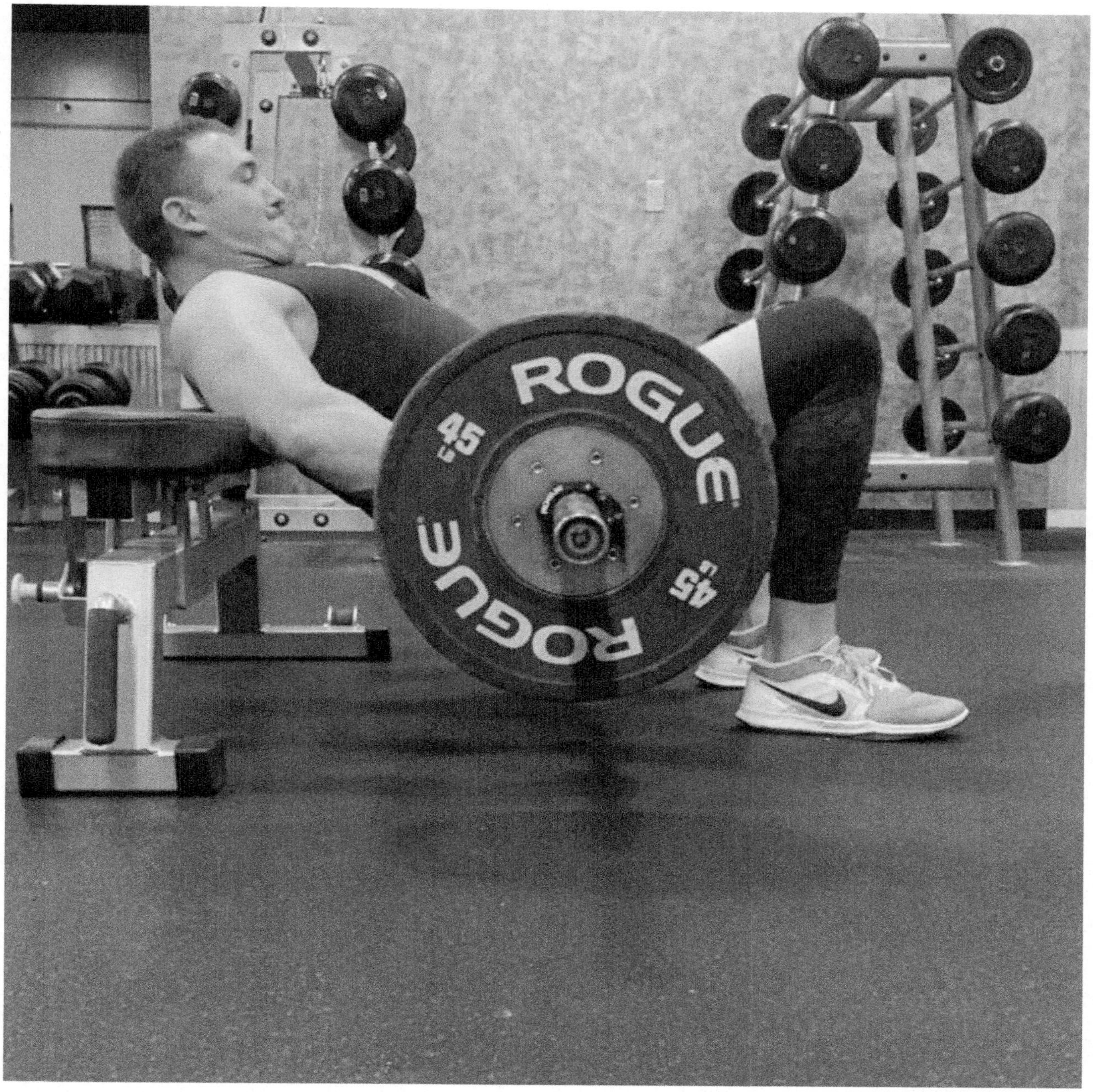

Pushing through the feet, the hips will extend up, squeezing the glutes at the top. The movement should be somewhat fast and violent.

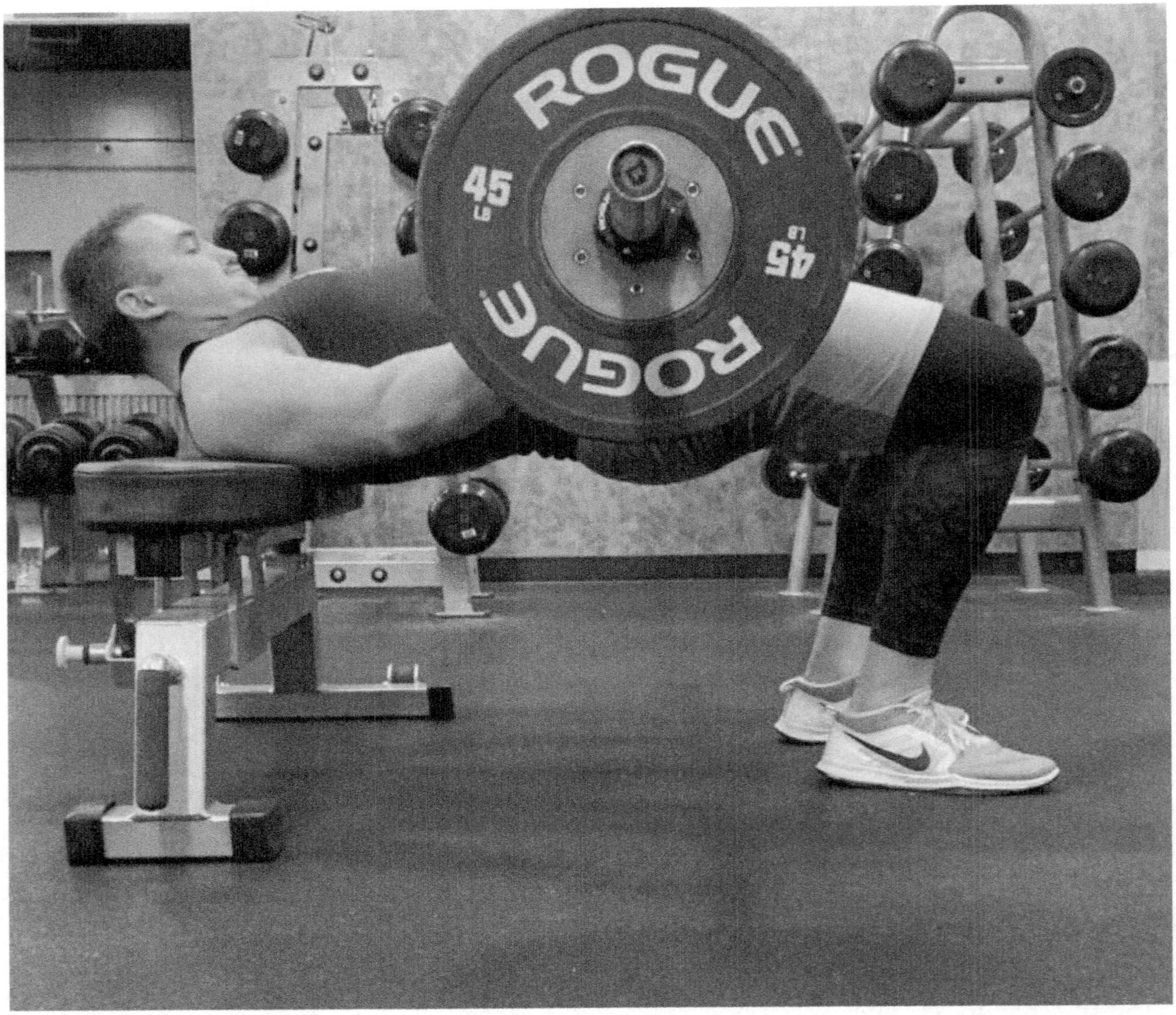

Push Jerk

Purpose:
A lot like the bench press, the push jerk is a great test of complete upper body strength and power. This is best described as an "Athletic Military Press." As coaches, we should aim for everything we do in the weight room to transfer onto the field of play. The push jerk is a great example of that. The primary muscle group being used is the Deltoids (shoulder), along with them, there are several secondary muscle groups including, but not limited to: triceps, biceps, core, quads and hamstrings. If we were to have opted for the traditional two dimensional lift in the military press, we would lose the transferable athletic element of this lift. Sure, you may target your deltoids a bit more, seeing how you have isolated them. However, sports do not require isolated movements.

Applies to the following Sport(s):
Various. Applies to sports that require the lower and upper body to work in unison with an explosive movement.

Applies to the following Position(s):
Various.

Equipment:
- Olympic sized Barbell
- Enough weight in varied sizes to supply and accommodate the strongest athlete
- Two safety clips for both ends of the bar
- A strong, sturdy rack or cage with adjustable bar racks and spotter racks
- A flat surface for the athlete to stand and perform lift

Spotter:

This lift will take place in a Rack or Cage, similar to a squat. The Push Jerk is going to require the athlete to push weight above their heads, which in turn can lead to serious, or even fatal injuries, spotting is a non-negotiable situation.

The Spotter will be standing behind the athlete performing the lift, with their hands up in a position to place on the scapulas. If the bar is in the air, and the athlete loses grip or fails, the spotter needs to be prepared to push the athlete forward to avoid the bar crashing on the skull, neck or back of the athlete.

It is always good to demonstrate all spotting technique especially with lifts like this one. Explain to the athlete that they do not need to push so hard that the push in itself will create an injury, but just hard enough to move their teammate out of danger.

Technique:

- Athletes will walk into the Rack towards the bar, and place hands at a shoulder grip or up to 6 inches outside of shoulders.
- With Hands spaced evenly apart, the athlete will place their shoulders under the bar with a solid grip.
- The athlete will then pick up the bar, take 1-2 steps back and place their feet under their hips. A stagger in the feet is also acceptable, but still only hip to hip distance.
- With a spotter present, the Athlete will start with a dip of the hips, and slight bend of the knees.
- From the bottom position, the athlete will explode the weight from chest to fully extended arms above the head.
- The athlete should have their head under the bar at the top of the lift while looking straight ahead.
- With simultaneous movement, the weight will now be lowered back to the chest, while the hips start to dip and knees start to bend, and repeat until the set is complete.

Max Out Procedure:

There is no Max Out for this lift. This is a lift that should be incorporated with push days, or upper body days as often as possible.

Alternated Lifts / Modification:

- Dumbbell / kettlebell push jerks
- Military Press (standing or seated)
- Handstand push-ups (prison pushups)

The feet should be under the hips. The hands should be placed right outside the shoulders.

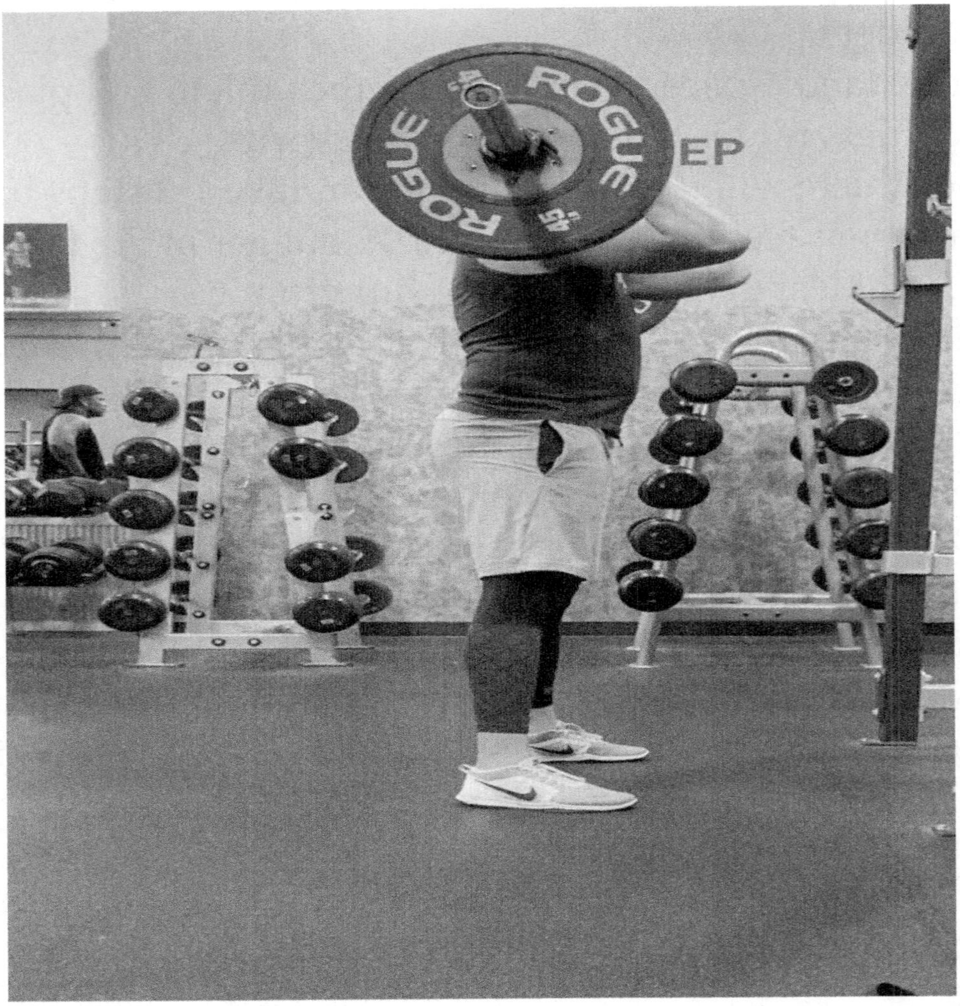

A slight knee bend should occur in order to perform the jerk portion of the lift.

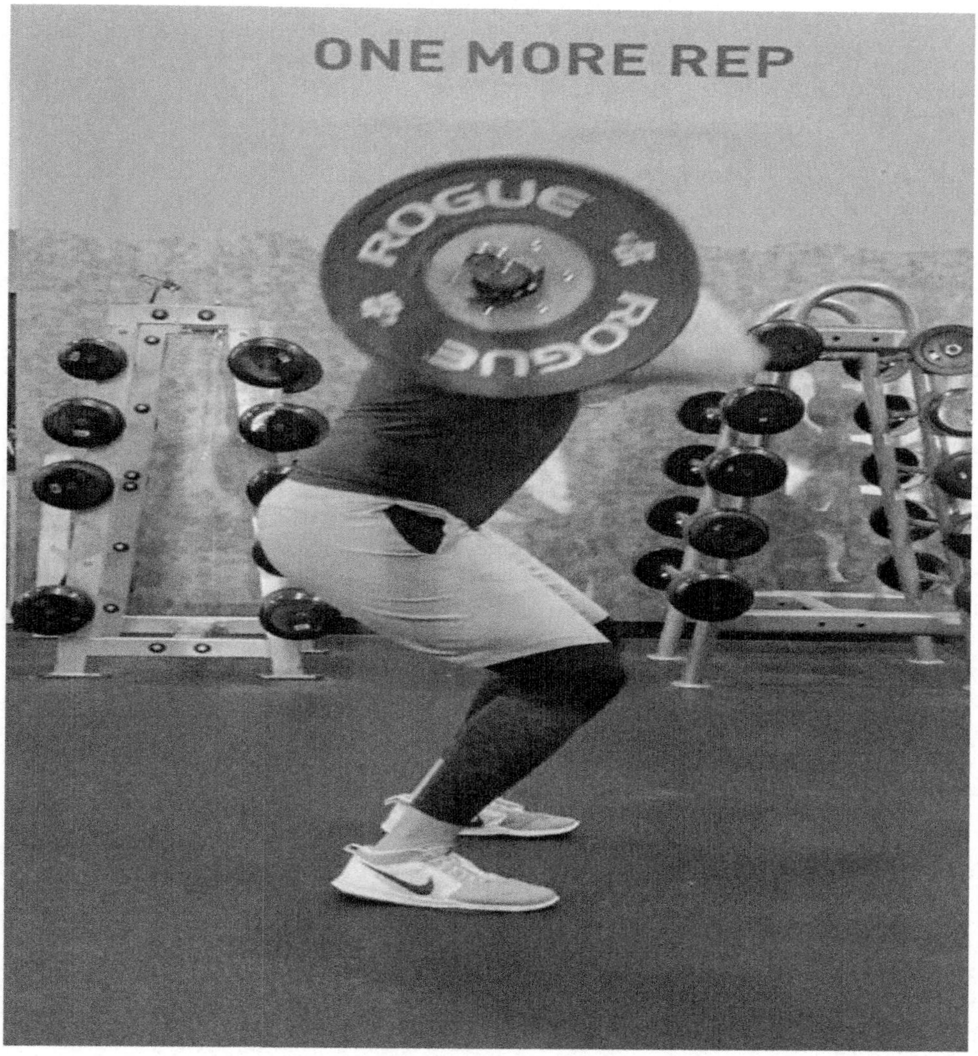

On the Press and Jerk it should happen as one fluid motion, pressing up violently through the toes.

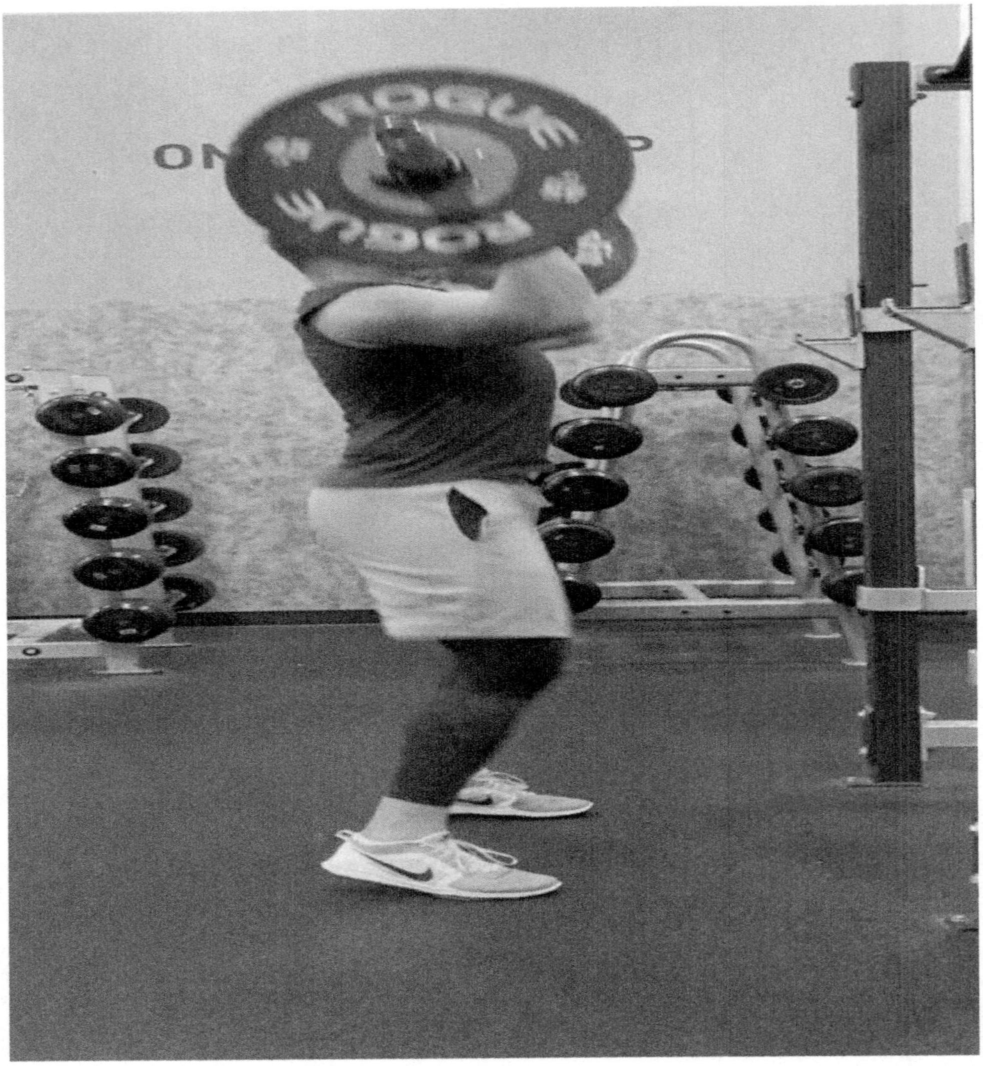

Finish with the head under the bar or "through the window" with a slight hip hinge and weight back on the heels.

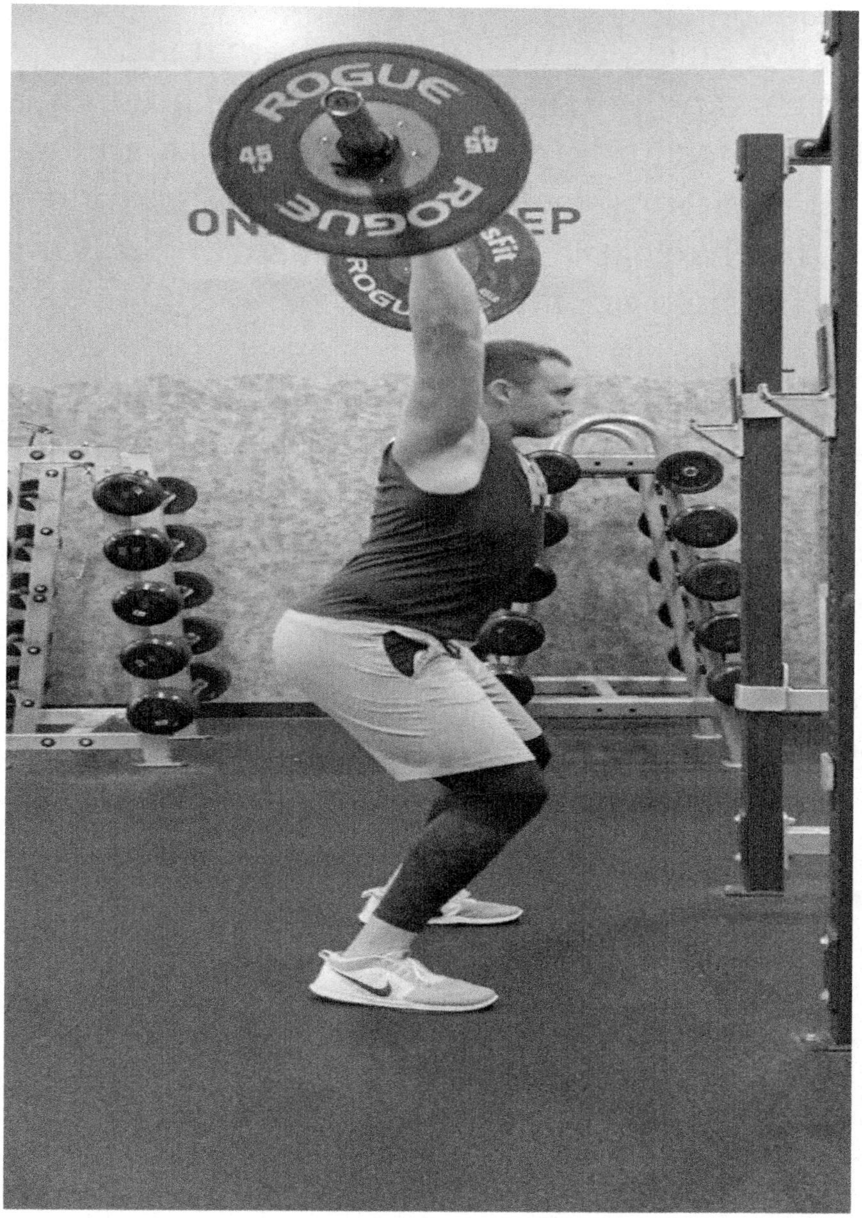

Hang Pull

Purpose:
The Hang Pull is an explosive movement, that is an integral part of the hang clean and power clean. It is the phase of the clean that leads into the snatch and drop phase. It is a fast, and violent movement. If done in an isolated movement, it would be an upright row, but like explained in the push jerk, it is important to transfer onto the field of play.

This lift should have a permanent spot in any program geared towards explosive athletes. It is especially great for football, and contact sport athletes because you are continually exerting great amounts of force to complete this lift, just like the athlete would during a competition.

Applies to the following Sport(s):
Various. Best suited for contact sport athletes and explosive athletics.

Applies to the following Position(s):
Various.

Equipment:

- Olympic sized Barbell
- Enough weight in varied sizes to supply and accommodate the strongest athlete
- Two safety clips for both ends of the bar
- A strong, sturdy rack or cage with adjustable bar racks and spotter racks
- A flat surface for the athlete to stand and perform lift

Spotter:

No spotter required. It is always advised to have a teammate watching, in the case of an emergency.

Technique:

- Like the Hang Clean, the athlete will start in a standing position holding the bar (power clean grip).
- Next, the Athlete will bring the bar down to the knee or right above the knee, brushing against the thigh while keeping the head and chest up, and pushing the hips and butt back.
- At this point the athlete is going to perform ONE fluid motion from above the knee to the top of the lift.
- The top of the lift should be:
    - Elbows up
    - The bar should be at the nipple line of the athlete
    - Hips forward
    - On their tippy toes
    - Scapulas squeezed together

Max Out Procedure:
There is no Max Out for this lift. This is a lift that should be incorporated with pull days, or upper body days as often as possible.

Alternated Lifts / Modification:

- Upright rows (Barbell, Dumbbell, Kettlebell)
- Kettlebell swings

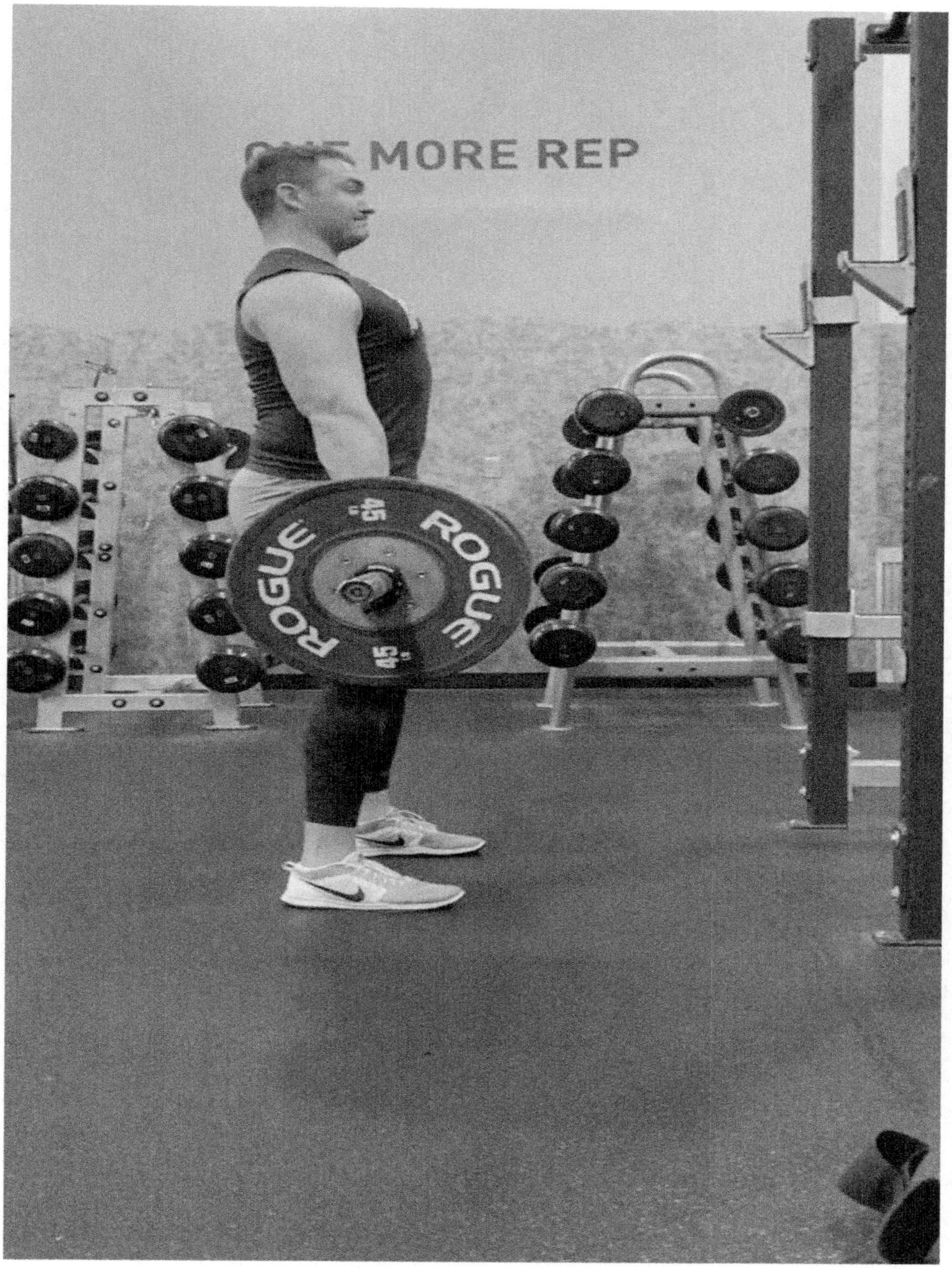
MORE REP
ROGUE
ROGUE
45

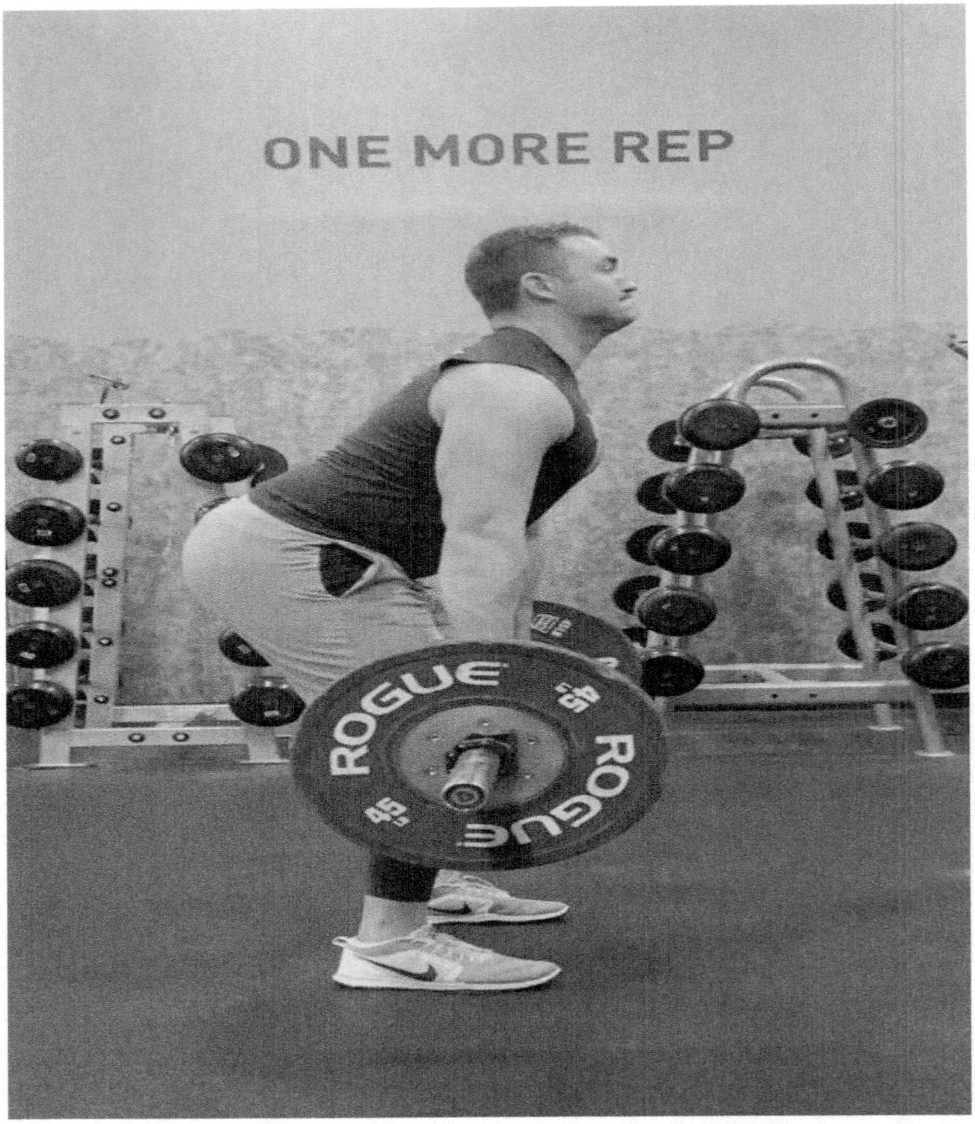
ONE MORE REP
ROGUE
ROGUE

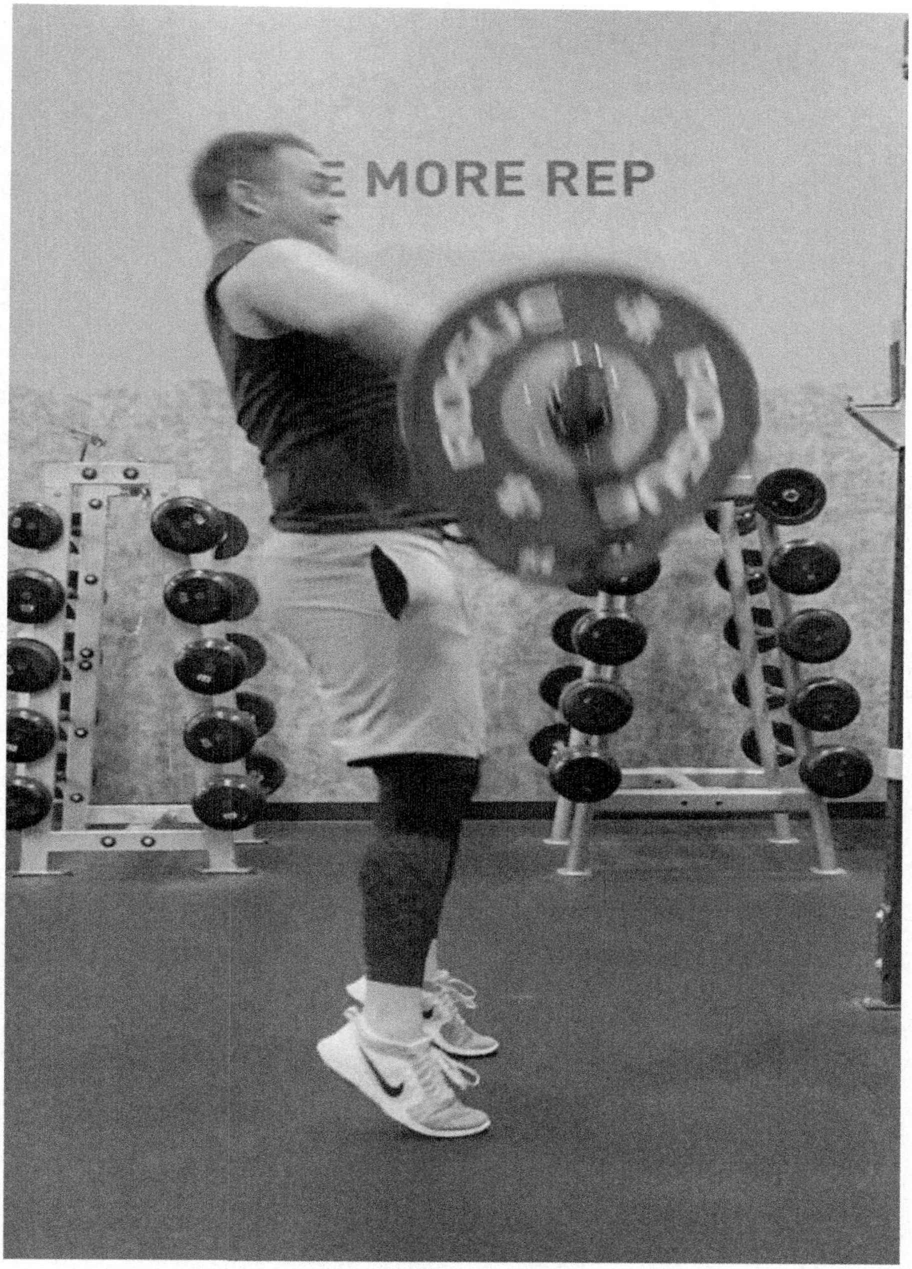
E MORE REP

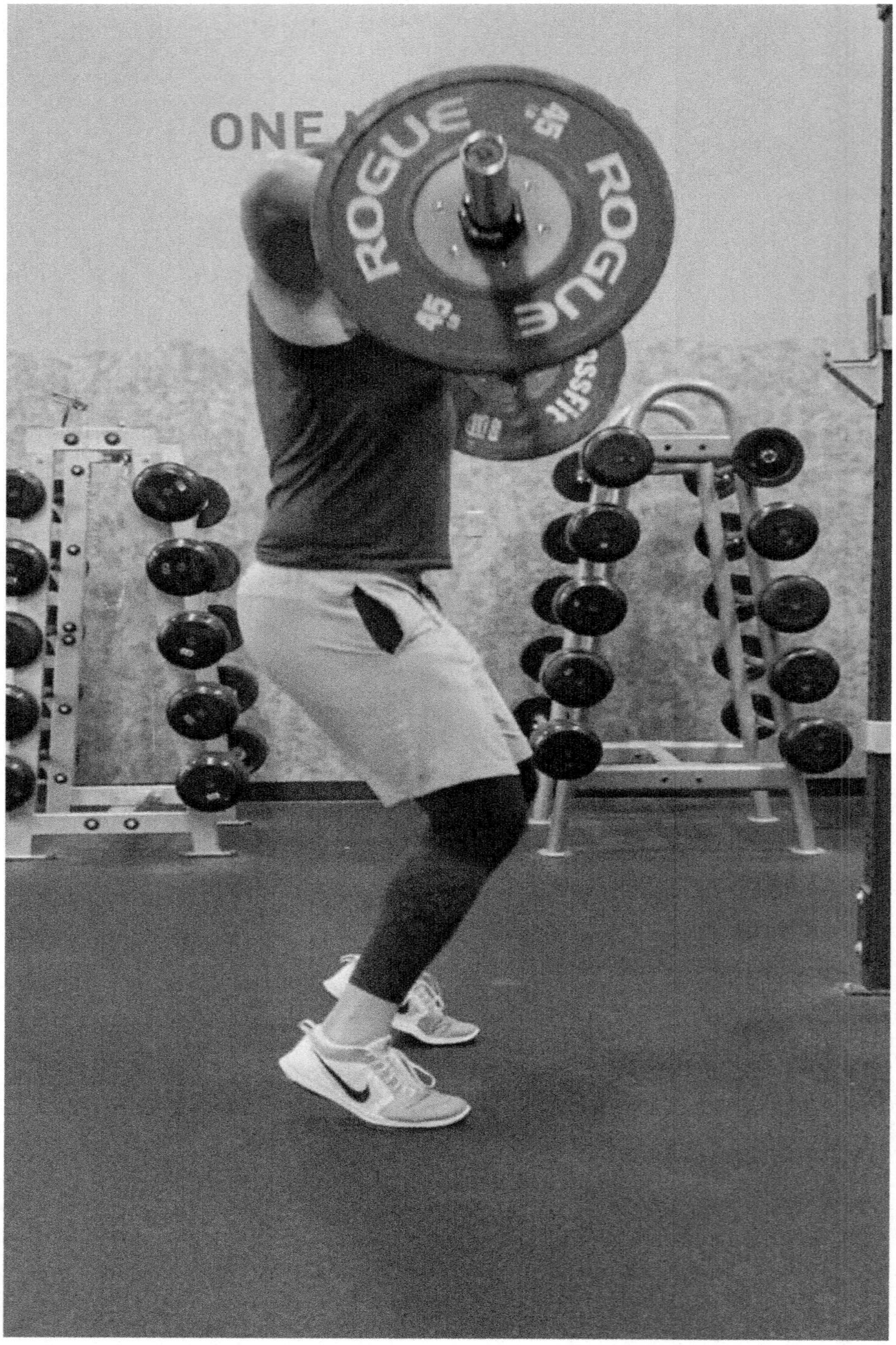
ONE
ROGUE
45
ROGUE
45

Power Pull

Purpose:
The Power Pull is an explosive movement that is an integral part of the power clean. It is the first phase of the clean; it is how the athlete should leave the ground with the bar. It is a fast and violent movement. If done in an isolated movement, it would be like performing a deadlift and doing a shrug after each rep. However, like explained in the Push Jerk and Hang Pull, we need it to transfer onto the field of play by making the lift athletic and functional.

This lift should have a permanent spot in any program geared towards explosive athletes. It is especially great for football, and contact sport athletes because you are continually exerting great amounts of force to complete this lift, just like the athlete would during a competition.

Applies to the following Sport(s):
Various. Best suited for contact sport athletes and explosive athletics.

Applies to the following Position(s):
Various.

Equipment:

- Olympic sized Barbell
- Enough weight in varied sizes to supply and accommodate the strongest athlete
- Two safety clips for both ends of the bar
- A strong, sturdy rack or cage with adjustable bar racks and spotter racks
- A flat surface for the athlete to stand and perform lift

Spotter:

No spotter required. It is always advised to have a teammate watching, in the case of an emergency.

Technique:

- The athlete needs to have their feet under or just outside of their hips.
- The athletes will place their hands just outside of their hips (feet if a little wide in their stance).
- The most important ques for the Athlete to follow will be to keep their chest and head up, butt down, and the bar against their legs.
- The Athlete needs to drive through their legs first.
- Once the bar is lifted off the ground and around the pelvic area, the athlete wants to drive the hips forward, while retracting their scapulas and shrugging their shoulders up in a violent fashion (hug their ears with their shoulders).
- Again, the athlete should finish the top of the lift with:
    - The bar against their body
    - On their tippy toes
    - Shoulders hugging their ears
    - Scapulas retracted
    - Hips forward
    - Head up

Max Out Procedure:

There is no Max Out for this lift. This is a lift that should be incorporated with pull days, or upper body days as often as possible.

Alternated Lifts / Modification:

- Shrugs (BB, DB, KB)
- Deadlifts (BB,DB,KB)

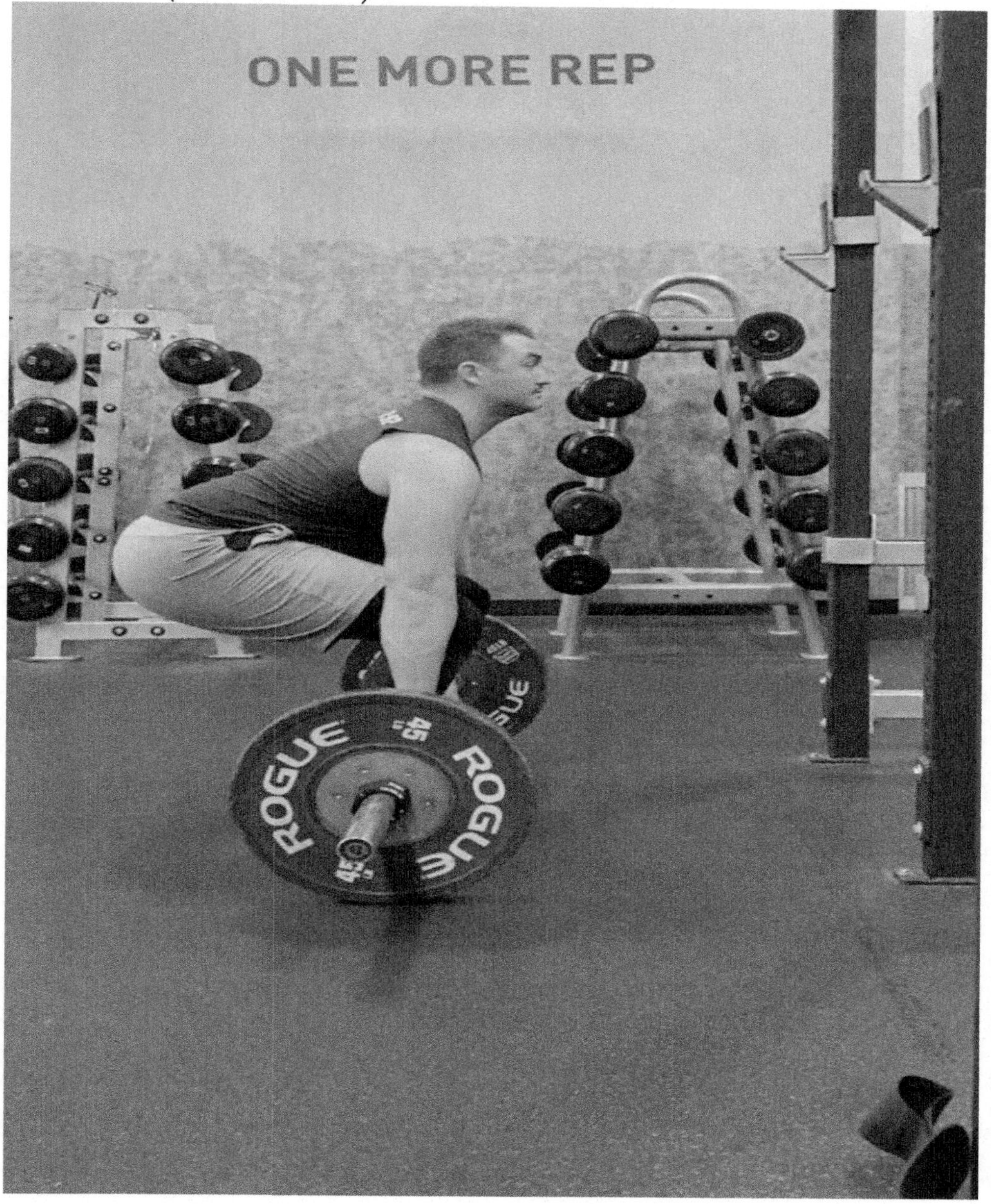

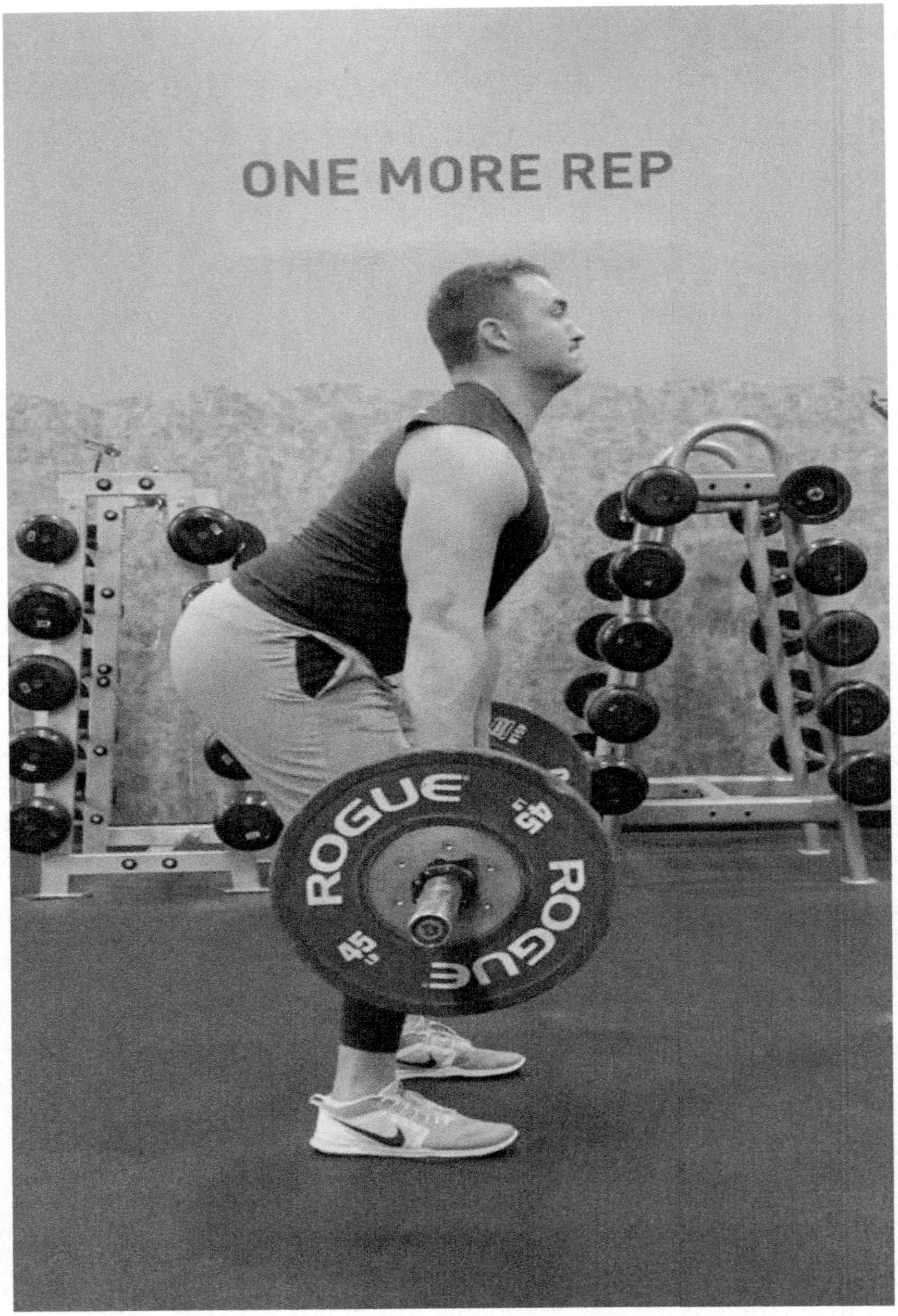
ONE MORE REP
ROGUE
45
ROGUE
45

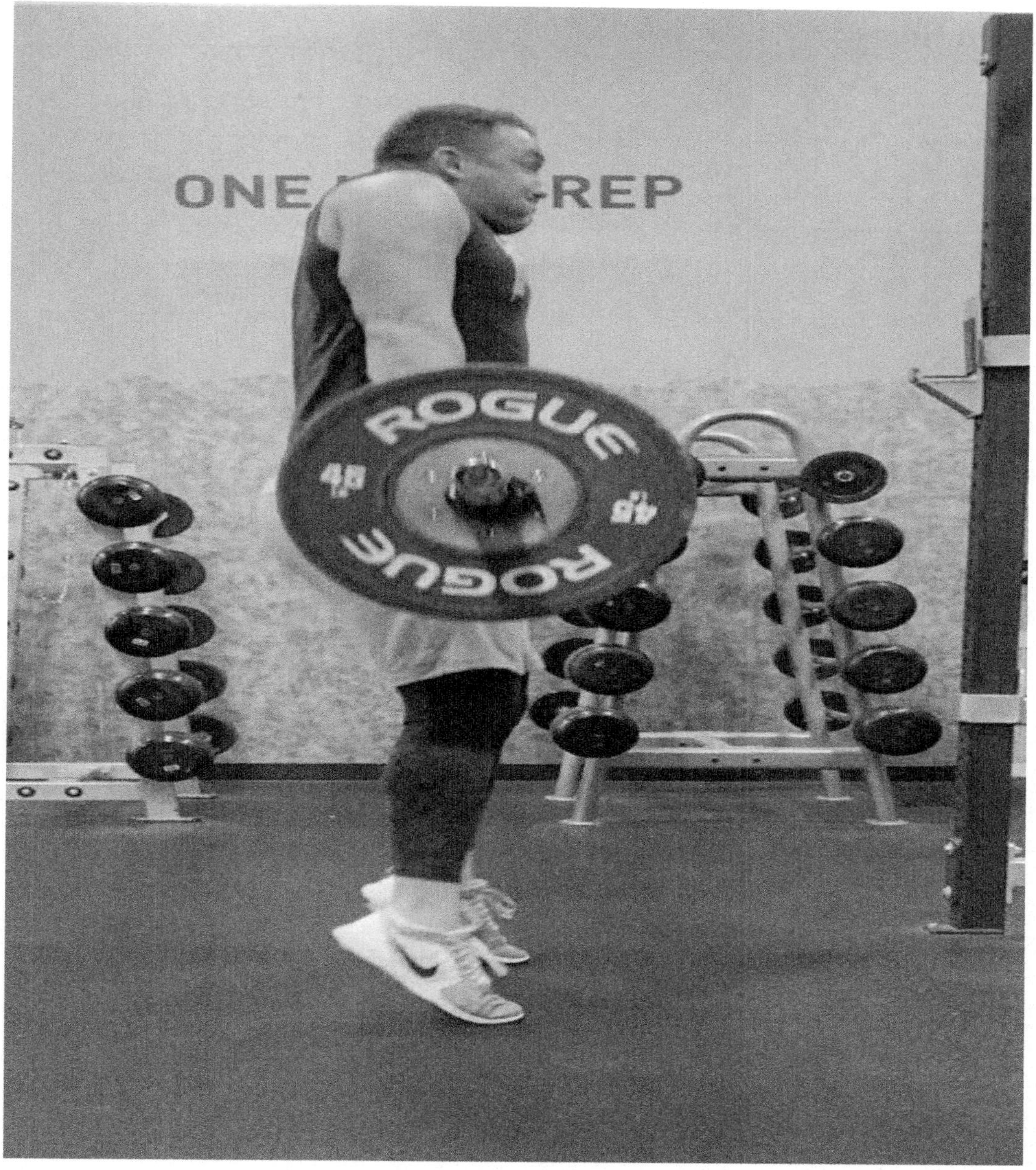

Finish with the hips forward, on the toes, the shoulders back and shrugging.

Reflection Notes:

Reflection Notes – Continued:

Reflection Notes – Continued:

Reflection Notes – Continued:

Chapter 4: Conditioning Procedures & Techniques

There are over 8,000 different sports in the world. The tests found in this chapter can be used across almost all sports when conditioning starts, like a universal language. The Pro Agility Test is one that all sports should be using. Followed by the Vertical and Board Jump. The 40-Yard Dash is one of the conditioning tests that is especially known for being used in the sport of football.

Here is just a small **List of Sports** that are well-known:

- Australian Football
- Baseball
- Basketball
- Cheerleading
- Cross Country
- Football (American Tackle)
- Golf
- Gymnastics
- Netball
- Rugby
- Soccer
- Softball
- Swimming
- Tennis
- Track
- Volleyball
- Wrestling

The Template of a Conditioning Test© will include:

Name of Conditioning Test – the Title

History:

Applies to the following Sport(s):

Applies to the following Position(s):

Equipment:

Recorder's Job:

Technique:

How often:

Things you can do to improve it:

40-Yard Dash

The **40-Yard Dash** is (36.58m) this is mainly tested to evaluate the speed and acceleration of an athlete, especially in American Tackle Football Players.

History:
This test originated with the average distance of a punt and the time it took to reach that distance. Back then an average hang time for a punt was around 4.5 seconds. So, the idea was, if a player could run that fast they could run from the line of scrimmage and catch a punt before it hits the ground; if it was punted straight.

Applies the following Sport(s):
Mainly just American Tackle Football

Applies to the following Position(s):
Every American Tackle Football Position

Equipment:

- About 8 cones or lines to mark off 40-yards
- A flat surface, like a track or field that has about 60-yards for deceleration and so they don't run into anything
- A timing system -- electronic laser timers are best and the most accurate; however, a stop watch will work but it does not provide as accurate of a reading

Recorder's Job:
There are many different ways to time this test when athletes are running the 40-yard dash. When a coach uses a thumb the time won't be as accurate as an electric timer.

Procedure:

- Dynamic Warm Up.
- Practice runs (2-3) at sub maximal speed.
- Use a three-point or 4-point sprinter stance so the athlete gets into a starting position.
- If using an electronic laser timer, the athlete may start when ready; if using a stopwatch, the athlete will start when given a cue.
- The average of two runs to the nearest tenth of a second is recorded.

How often:

This is like a Fitnessgram test. You do it only a couple times a season and you only have athletes do it twice in the same day.

Things you can do to improve it:

Certain aspects of speed training are often overlooked and can be a slow developing process. When we think of athletes that demonstrate speed we often think of track and field athletes that are oftentimes just born fast; the gift they possess cannot be taught.

The following are a few things that can help an athlete get faster:

- Lifting weights/Resistance Training.
- Heavy/deep squats, resistance training with knee drives, hip mobility.
- Mechanics training:
    - Repetitive training of sprinting mechanics
    - Muscle Memory is key
    - It requires 3,000-5,000 reps for muscle memory to really kick in.

Pro Agility (5-10-5)

"The Pro Agility Test should be the test that the majority of coaches use to measure an athlete's ability to perform short speed burst and Cut on a Dime (COD)." -- Coach Stone

This drill is designed to measure short-area quickness, lateral movement, flexibility & the speed at which a player can change directions on a moment's notice. The drill also gives coaches an idea on whether or not the athlete can stay low as well as demonstrate their ability to sink their hips and get up and go.

History:
This test is one of those that you can't find who invented but if you look really hard you can find that it was used as a protocol outlined by Harmann et al. (1).

Applies to the following Sport(s):
Every Sport

Applies to the following Position(s):
Every Position

Equipment:

- 3 cones per athlete
- 20-yards of running space and another 10-yards to left or right -- outside of the area.
- Some kind of stopwatch or a way to record the time. Electronic laser timers are best, and the most accurate; however, a stop watch will work with not as accurate a reading.

Recorder's Job:
The athlete will align in the middle of the 10-yard mark. On movement, they will go either left or right. Make sure to emphasize to the athlete that they should run all the way through the last cone to make sure they run their best time.

Procedure:

- Dynamic Warm Up.
- Practice runs (2-3) at sub maximal speed.
- Using a three-point even stance, the athlete will either go right or left for 5-yards, then change direction for 10-yards, with one more change of direction for 5-yards.
- The athlete's foot must touch each line.
- Make sure to explain to the athlete that they will face forward the entire time, including every Change of Direction (If they choose to go left, they will touch the first line with their left hand, when going right, they will touch the line with their right hand.)
- If using an electronic laser timer, the athlete may start when ready; if using a stopwatch, the athlete will start when given a cue.
- The average of two runs to the nearest tenth of a second is recorded.

How often:
This is like a Fitnessgram test. Only do it a couple times a season and only have athletes do it twice in the same day. You should do this test going both left and right at least once each time or twice.

Things you can do to improve it:

- Lifting weights/ Resistance Training.
- Heavy/deep squats, resistance training with knee drives, hip mobility.
- Mechanics training:
    - Repetitive training of sprinting mechanics
    - Muscle Memory is key
    - It requires 3,000-5,000 reps for muscle memory to really kick in.

Vertical Jump

History:
Some sources say this standard test for measuring the vertical jump is called the "**Sargent Jump Test"** (First tested in 1921), which was invented by **Dr. Dudley Sargent** approximately 90 years ago. This test is the act of jumping straight up into the air. This is an effective exercise for building both endurance and explosive power. Coaches say this is a standard test for measuring the power output of an athlete.

Applies to the following Sport(s):
All Sports

Applies to the following Position(s):
All Positions

Equipment:
- You can use a wall with measurement markers on it. Have the athlete do the Vertical testing poll (seen at the NFL combine)
- Just Jump Pad (electronic pad that measures vertical jumping ability)

Recorder's Job:
Depends on the equipment being used.
- Record the athlete's reach. (Pre-Jump, the athlete stands vertical and lifts arm up as high as possible. Measure Inches touched.)
- When an athlete jumps, take the jump number and the reach number and subtract them to get the vertical number.

Technique:

- WITHOUT taking a stutter step, the athlete can perform a countermovement by flexing at the hips and knees (like we train in the weight room).
- On the jump up, the hips should be driven forward, while the dominant hand reaches up towards the marker, and the non-dominant hand drives down.

How often:

This is like a Fitnessgram test. Only do it a couple times a season and only have athletes do it twice in the same day.

Things you can do to improve it:

- Lifting weights / Resistance Training.
- Heavy/deep squats, resistance training with knee drives, hip mobility.
- Mechanics training:
    - Repetitive training of sprinting mechanics
    - Muscle Memory is key
    - It requires 3,000-5,000 reps for muscle memory to really kick in.

Broad Jump

History:
The Broad Jump originated as a jumping event in track and field. Until 1912, it was an event in the olympics. Nowadays, it is commonly practiced for competition in the NFL combine.

Applies to the following Sport(s):
All Sports

Applies to the following Position(s):
All Positions

Equipment:

- Lines measured out on a flat surface reaching up to 12-15 Feet.

Recorder's Job:

- To measure the heel line of the athlete after a clean jump (toes start behind the line, stuck the landing without falling or moving feet) is performed.

Technique:

- The athlete will need to create a countermovement by swinging both arms back and forth, while hips are also going forward to backward simultaneously.
- The athlete will make the jump while thrusting their hips and hands in the direction of the jump.
- The athlete will need to land into the jump (a squatting position) to help stick the landing without falling or moving their feet.

How often:
This is like a Fitnessgram test. Only do it a couple times a season and only have athletes do it twice in the same day.

Things you can do to improve it:

- Lifting weights / Resistance Training.
- Heavy/deep squats, resistance training with knee drives, hip mobility.
- Mechanics training:
    - Repetitive training of sprinting mechanics
    - Muscle Memory is key
    - It requires 3,000-5,000 reps for muscle memory to really kick in.

Reflection Notes:

Reflection Notes – Continued:

Reflection Notes – Continued:

Reflection Notes – Continued:

Chapter 5:
Speed and PlyoMetric Training

Speed -- The rate (or time) it takes an object to move a certain distance.

Speed Training is the cumulative sum of several different training aspects. Such as, resistance training (weight lifting), sprinting technique, and muscular flexibility.

Speed is most often determined by the athlete's ability to apply a vast quantity of force in a short period of time, or more simply known as power. An athlete that can produce the most force in the shortest amount of time is going to be the most effective.

Resistance Training increases an athlete's maximal force production. As a result of resistance training the athlete can produce more force and can do so in the same period of time; as a result, strength training can increase the athlete's power. However, it is important for the strength coach to develop the "Whole" athlete as best as possible. That is why it is best to increase both maximal force production and the rate of force. This can be achieved through training techniques that increase the athletes power, some of those are plyometrics training, and variations of lifts that produce power like power cleans, squatting with depth, and speed on the way up. Both strength and power training are absolutely necessary to improve an athlete's speed.

Proper Sprinting Mechanics is as important an aspect of becoming faster as anything else. Everything from the first step, to the stride, the arm movement, the body lean, and even breathing. If you are not familiar with the importance of these mechanics then refer to someone experienced in this area, like a

Track Coach. If you do not have access to a Track Coach then research the topic and look for valid resources on the Internet.

When it comes time to condition your team, take that opportunity to have them participate in speed drills and drills that emphasize agility, quickness, speed, and change of direction. Conditioning should be limited to drills that will translate to Game Day.

Example: During competition, a football player rarely ever runs 110-yards. So, why run a 110-yards during conditioning? It isn't improving their Speed. It doesn't translate to competition. What happens is it breaks the athlete's sprinting form.

Conditioning drills that are good, 5-10-5 Pro Shuttle, any sprints within 40-50 yards, then the big fellas should be capped at 40. Sideline to sideline (Stride from sideline to hash, sprint from hash to hash, back to stride to sideline) this is great practice for the athlete changing their velocity during competition. Anything that can be related to what a player does in a game, with the competition related rest periods, will be great for conditioning and speed training.

Plyometric Training is a type of jump training, in simple terms. The goal of Plyometric Training is to increase power by having the athlete exert maximal force in short periods of time. Plyos are something that can be added to all programs with the purpose to increase an athlete's power. Doing this allows the athlete to run faster, get up in the air higher, and accomplish (COD) Change of Direction faster. These movements also prepare the body for the type of impact and environment it encounters during competition, which should lead to a decrease in injury.

Speed Endurance Drills
Speed, It Is The Name Of The Game.

Speed is a necessary attribute in today's game. When we look at our best players, and the players we see playing on Saturdays, Sundays, and Monday nights, the common denominator is speed. While we watch the NFL combine we watch blazing 40 times, and they just get faster every year. In today's game we have 6'4+ 300+ pound offensive and defensive lineman running 4.4- 4.6 40-yard dashes, which is absolutely insane.

The game requires it. Offenses want to spread out and use all 53 ⅓ yards. They want to use screens, jet sweeps, outside zones, and all of these things that stretch the field and require all athletes to possess some speed, including the big fellas. Defenses need to find a way to match that, so pass rushers need great speed, because the passing games are becoming quick, no more 7 step drops and rarely are there 5 step drops. Offenses want the ball in the hands of these speedy playmakers as soon as possible.
The truth about speed is, only a fraction of athletes are genetically wired to be fast. They have those fast twitch muscle fibers that are hard wired in their makeup, and not everybody is created equally in the speed game. Can we develop athletes to get faster? Yes. Can we develop athletes to get quicker? Yes. If a player is slow, can we develop them to be fast? Probably not. They either have it or they don't. I know that is a harsh reality, but it is in most cases at least, it is the truth. The best we can do is develop their mechanics, increase their strength & mobility, giving them the tools necessary to become as fast as they possibly can.

Additional Ways to Work with Players on Increasing Their Speed (If available):

- Run Up and Down Stairs or Stadium Stairs
- Run in the Sand
- Run in the Swimming Pool
- Swimming: 10 Laps Freestyle, 10 Laps Backstroke, 10 Laps Side Stroke

Coaching Tip: **Use the Dynamic Stretches (FWU) for your Every Day Stretches.**

Dynamic Stretches (FWU)
Functional Warm Up

1) Walking High Knees
2) Forward Lunge
3) Backward Lunge
4) Slow Shuffle (SUMOS)
5) Quick High Knees
6) Butt Kicks
7) Quick Carioca
8) Quick Shuffle
9) Tin Soldiers
10) 123 Touch
11) Crazy Legs
12) Carioca

Agile Bag Drills

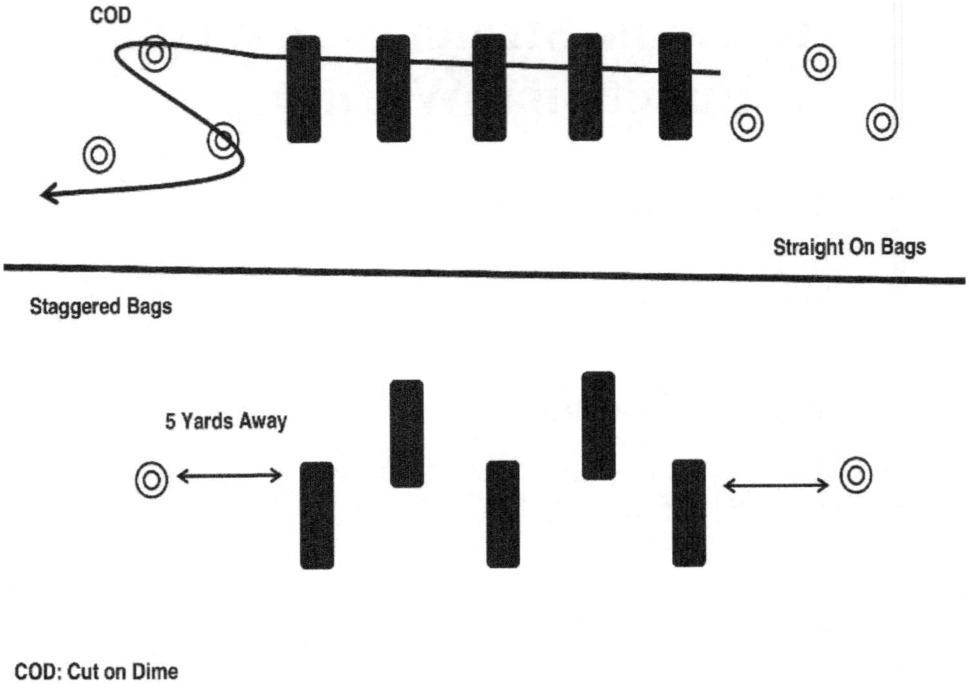

Straight Bags – 2 reps each direction (see the diagram on the previous page):

1) Jog Straight
2) High Knees
3) Bunny Hops
4) Slalom Hops
5) In/Out Drill
6) Lateral Step Thru
7) Stride (Older Players)
8) Finish: Sprint through 5-yards
9) Finish: COD (Cut on Dime) -- 3 Cones

Stagger Bags – 2 reps each direction (see the diagram on the previous page):

1) Vertical Quick Step
2) Lateral Quick Step
3) Finish: Sprint through 5 yards or COD (3) Cones

Coaching Points:

- Keep Eyes up – Coach will show numbers to make sure players keep their eyes up.
- Stay low, in good posture
- Pump Arms
- Lateral Drills – run over bags, face coach, never cross feet

Modification:
Add a football once players master the above drills.

Note: Most players tend to get too high during the bags. Bag drills teach players to get their feet over fallen bodies while keeping their eyes on the backfield action.

More Agile Bag Drills

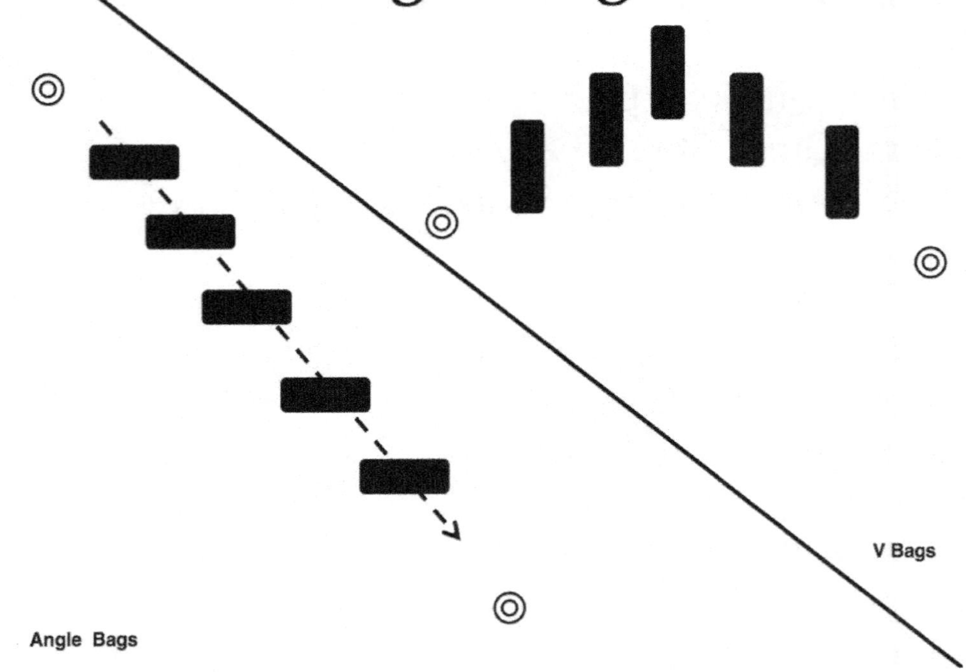

Angle Bags – 2 reps each direction (Some Speed Drills are geared toward Defense):

1) Downhill COD on Coach
   a. Coach Points which direction the player should Run
   b. Don't slow down
2) Downhill with a Cut Ball (Older Players) (Offense and Defense)
   a. Player runs downhill, coach throws cut ball
3) Downhill with Hand Shield (Coach Holding at end) (Offense and Defense)
   a. Player runs downhill and uses a hand shield
4) Downhill with Boot Action (Offense and Defense)
   a. Player runs downhill, coach boots away when player gets to the end

V Bags – 2 reps each direction:

1) Uphill / Reverse Pivot / Downhill / COD or Defeat a Block
2) Uphill / Reverse Pivot / Downhill / COD or Catch a Football

Coaching Points:

- Keep Eyes up – Coach will show numbers to make sure players keep their eyes up.
- Stay Low, in good posture
- Pump Arms
- Lateral Drills – run over bags, face coach, never cross feet

Modification:

Add a football once players master the above drills.

Note: Most players tend to get too high during the bags. Bag drills teach players to get their feet over fallen bodies while keeping their eyes on the backfield action.

Ladders

Ladders improve a player's agility, coordination, foot speed, and overall speed. There are numerous options on how to use ladders to condition a player; for example, have the players go down and back, or make it a maze where players go down one ladder and then up another ladder.

Different ways to do the Down and Back Drills

1) Both Feet	**6) Crazy Legs**	**11) Side Step**
2) Every other foot – start with the left foot and then the right foot	**7) Hips**	**12) Zig-Zag**
3) Jump – Feet together	**8) Slalom**	**13) High Knee**
4) Alternate Feet – Every other Foot	**9) In / Out**	**14) Bunny Hops**
5) Opposite Foot – start with the right foot and then the left foot	**10) Shuffle**	

Coaching Points:

- Keep Eyes up – Coach will show numbers to make sure players keep their eyes up.
- Stay Low, in good posture
- Pump Arms

Ropes

If your organization can store and/or afford the "old school" ropes we highly recommend them. There are multiple ways to use them.

Coaching Tip: Make sure they are 6 inches off the ground.

You can use almost all of the same ladder exercises with ropes, as well as the three shown below in the diagram.

Ropes

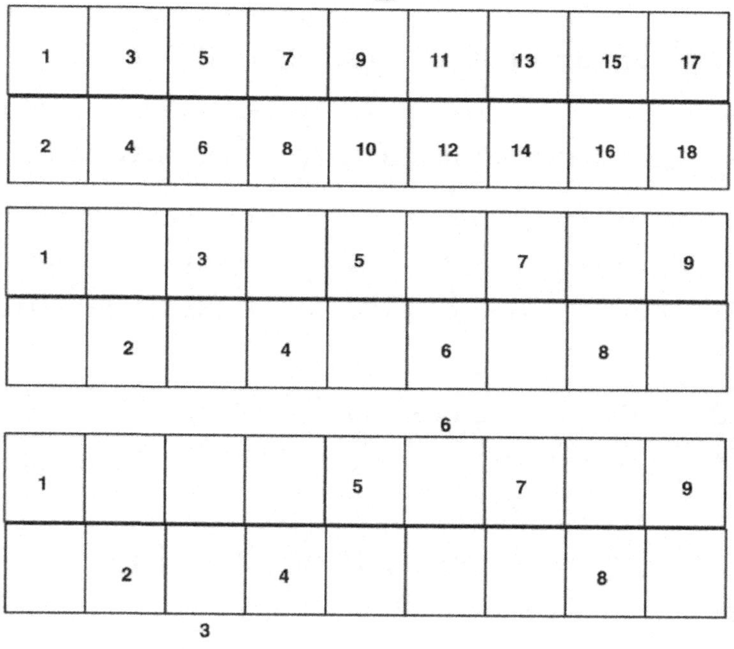

Jump Rope

Jumping Rope is the easiest and most effective exercise that every player must do. A player's performance will improve with Jumping Rope because it does the following: works every muscle, increases stamina, improves agility, improves balance, increases hand-eye coordination, and increases a player's speed. The following is how to incorporate a jump rope in your workout:

Jump rope for Speed

- Legs (100 Times) forward then backwards
- Left Leg (50 Times) forward then backwards
- Right Leg (50 Times) forward then backwards
- Start with the jump rope going as fast as possible for 10 seconds and count it – Do this at least three times
- When mastered going fast for 10 seconds then go as Fast as Possible for 30 seconds – 3x reps while someone else counts
- Crossover – 10x in a row without missing
- When mastered doing Crosses increase to 25 times without missing for 30 seconds.

Hop Over a Cone for Speed

This is a very basic but effective drill.

NOTE: Once a player goes over a cone they must come back to the beginning before going on to the next cone.

This drill increases a player's balance and agility. The following are the different ways to hop:

1) Two Legs Together
2) Left Leg
3) Right Leg

Hop over a cone for speed

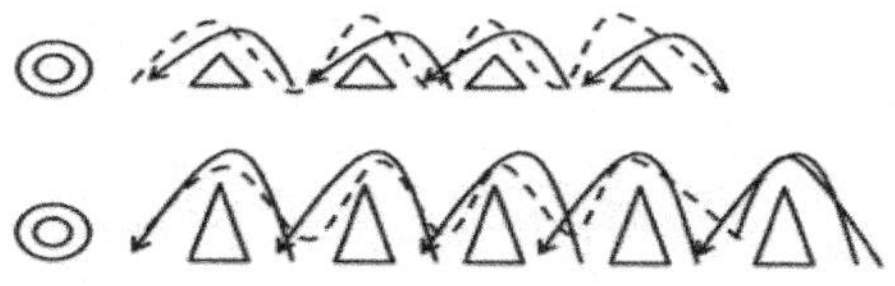

Cone Drills

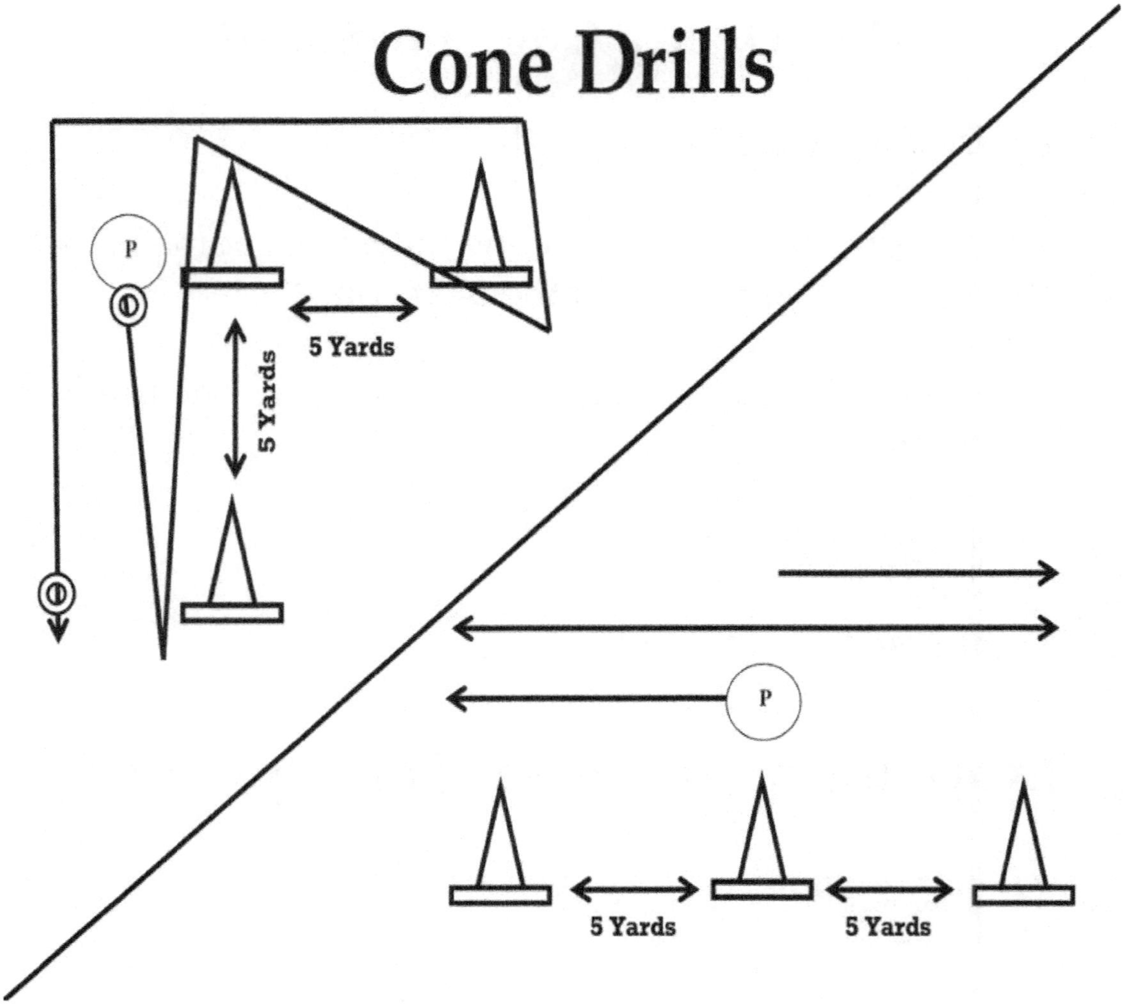

Cone Drills

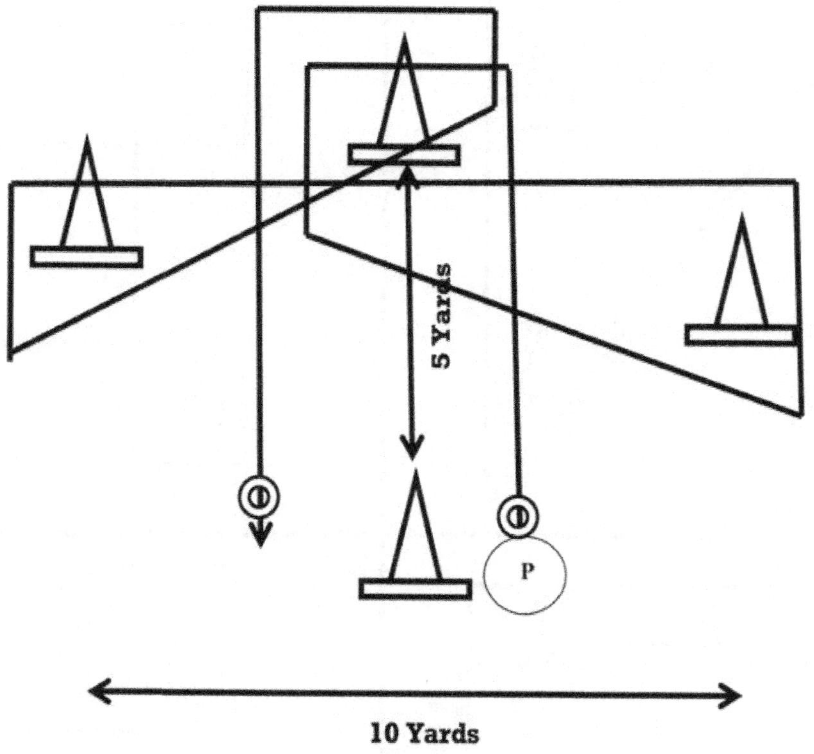

Cone Drills

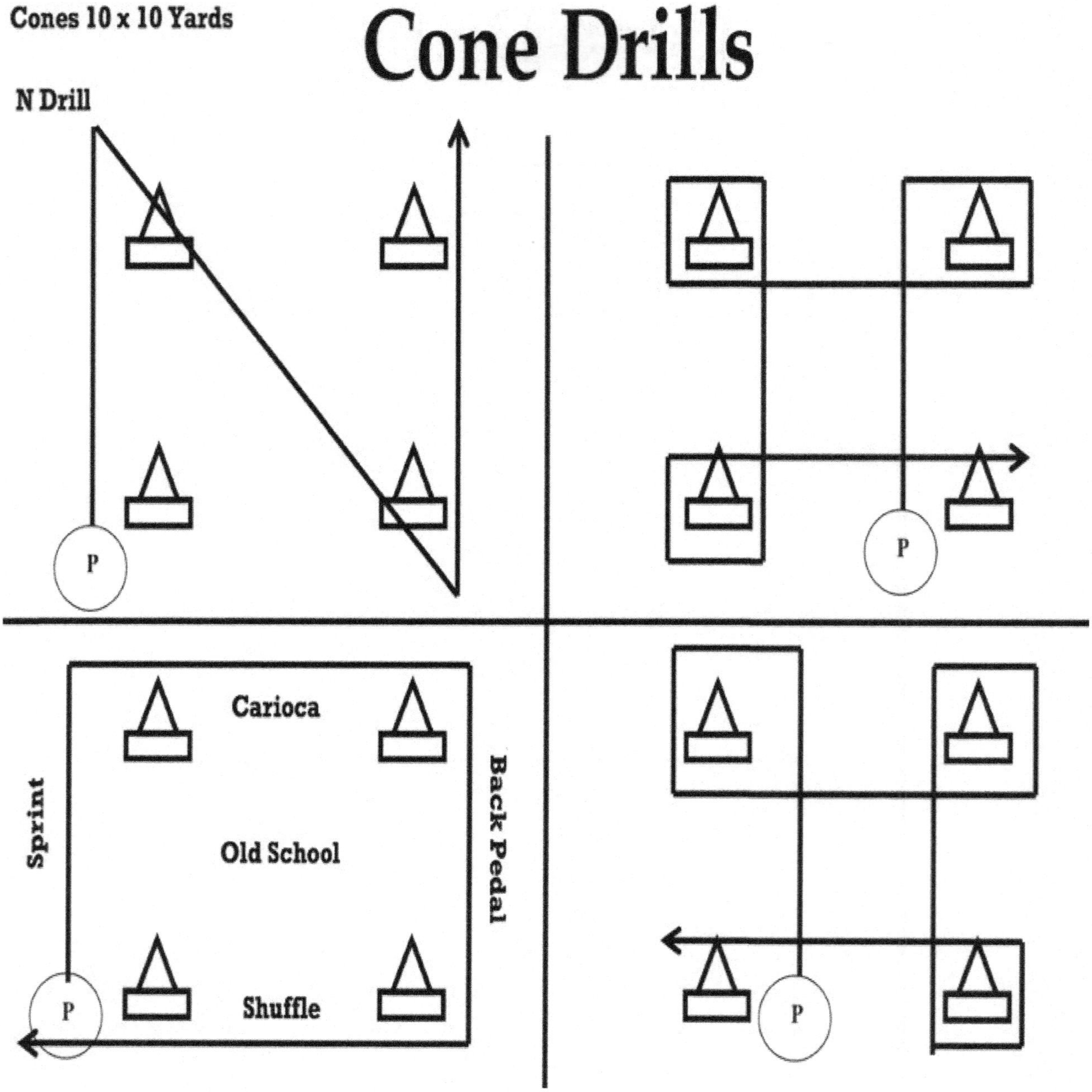
Cones 10 x 10 Yards
N Drill
P
P
Carioca
Sprint
Old School
Back Pedal
P
Shuffle
P

Reflection Notes:

Reflection Notes – Continued:

Reflection Notes – Continued:

Reflection Notes – Continued:

Chapter 6:
15-Minute Workouts (At Home / Travel)

Disclaimer: Please discuss working out in more detail with your Doctor, Athletic Trainer, or Team Doctor. Coach Stone and Coach Casazza are both firm believers in having players workout at home to help maintain the overall well being of their body in orderto stay in playing shape. Always take physical restrictions into consideration before advising a player to do a specific stretch or drill. We are not doctors and do not assume responsibility. We are just sharing effective ways to stretch a specific area. Please understand the stretches thoroughly and give proper instruction when directing players.

Example: Home Gym due to Covid-19 Restrictions

Monday UPPER:

- Dynamic Warmup
- 3-way Push-Ups: diamond, shoulder, wide -- 3 x 30 (10 each way)
- Dips -- 4 x 10 – failure (use the corners of what or a counter, or you can use a couch or chair)
- Prison Push-Ups -- 4 x 8-10 (feet on couch, bend over like you are doing a handstand. This should mimic an upside-down shoulder press)
- Curls -- 4 x 10-20 (use what you have: Barbell, dumbbells, bands, a chair, brick, rocks…)
- 3-way Planks -- 3 x 1 minute each way
- V-Ups -- 3 x 10
- Static Stretch

Tuesday LOWER:

- Dynamic Warmup
- Body Squats -- 4 x 20
- Walking Lunges -- 4 x 15 each leg
- Step Ups -- 4 x 10 each leg (drive the knee to the chest)
- Side Lunge -- 4 x 10 each way
- Falling Hamstring Curls -- 4 x 8
- Static Stretch

Wednesday SPEED TRAINING:

- Dynamic Warmup
- 10 x 10-yard Sprints
- 10 x 10-yard Power Skips
- 10 x 20-yard Hill Sprints
- 10 Practice Starts (focus on the first 2-3 steps working on the drive)
- Static Stretch

Thursday UPPER-

- Dynamic Warmup
- Pull-Ups -- 4 x 10
- Spiderman Push-Ups -- 4 x 10
- Inverted Rows -- 4 x 10
- Shoulder Circuit -- 3 x 30 secs. each way (straight arms the whole time) flutters palms out, flutters palms back, flutters palms down, half circles pronate/supinate, raise the roof)
- Pick 3 AB workouts -- do them 3 times each
- Static Stretch

Friday LOWER-

- Dynamic Warmup
- Squat Jumps -- 4 x 10
- Tuck Jumps -- 4 x 20 secs
- Broad Jumps -- 4 x 10
- Lunge Jumps -- 4 x 10 each leg
- Lateral Jumps to Sprints -- 4 x 10 each leg
- Single Leg Hops -- 4 x 20 sec
- Static Stretch

Below is a list of exercises that can be used to replace existing lifts after a 2-4 week duration. Remember, in times like today with COVID-19, we will not always have access to our weight facilities. Some might not even have access to a weight room to begin with it. Either way, equipment does not define the athlete; be resourceful and use what you have.

Here are a few reminders:

- More does not always equal better.

- If you are implementing something, have a reason for it. Do not just do something, to do it.

- Making a player sore is not necessarily a good thing. That does not mean it was a good workout.

- Always explain the "WHY" to a player. What is the reason behind an exercise or drill that you are having them do?

- Periodization!!!!!! Muscles need to repeat motions and actions several times to get something from it. Do not change up workouts every week. Lifts should change every 2-4 weeks at most. The intensity can change however.

Upper Body

Push-Ups
Bent Push-Ups
Sit-Ups
V-Ups
Crunches
Bicycles
Leg Lifts
Seated Triceps
Dips (If possible)
Seated (Chair) Triceps
Dumbbell Press (If you have dumbbells)
Dumbbell Rows
Side Bends
Dumbbell Side Bends
Bear Crawl
Alligator Crawl
Crab Crawl
Inchworm
Power Punch
Dumbbell Cross Jab
Uppercut
Jump Cross
Altering Renegade Row
Single-Arm Renegade Row
Single-Leg Renegade Row
Single-Arm T Row
Bench Dips
Triceps Dips
Assisted Bench Dip
Roller Triceps Dip
Single-Leg Bench Dip

Floor Dip
Single-Leg Floor Dip
Dip to Kick

Lower Body

Glute Bridge
Single-Leg Glute Bridge
Squat Jumps
Single-Leg Kickbacks
Side Kicks
Fire Hydrants
Jumping Jacks
Jumps
Side to Side
Forward and Backwards
Side Lying Hip Abduction
Side Lying Hip Adduction
Calf Raises
Single Leg Stand
Forward Lunge
Forward Lunge with Twist
Straight-Leg Lunge
Jumping Lunges
Walking Lunge
Dumbbell Walking Lunge
Reach and Twist Walking Lunge
Reverse Lunge
Lateral Lunge
Side Lunge Stretch
Toe Touches (Forward Bend)
Left Over Right Toe Touches
Right Over Left Toe Touches
Feet Wide Half Forward Bend
Alternating Toe Touches
Seated Toe Touches (Forward Bend)
Single Leg Seated Toe Touches (Forward Bend)

Donkey Kicks
Donkey Whips
Jumping
Distance Leap
Jump to Balance Ball
Cheer Jump
Depth Jumps
Tuck Jumps

Total Body

Running
Jogging
Skipping
Backpedaling
Butt Kicks
Farmer's Walk
Monster Walk
High Knees
Planks (Forearm & Upward)
Forearm Plank
- Forearm Plank Knee Drops
- Chaturanga (Low Plank)
- Spiderman Plank
- Arm-Reach Plank
- Plank-Up
- High Plank
- High Plank with Leg Extension
- High Plank Knee Pull-in
- Plank Roll Down

Upward Plank
Upward Plank Kicks
Upward Plank Hip Lift
Lateral Planks Walks
Side Planks
Forearm Planks
T-Stabilization
Kneeling Side Kick
Downward Facing Dog
Lateral Leg Raises
High Knees
Hug High Knees

Spider Mountains Climbers
Mountain Climbers
Stretches
Wall Sits
Lunges (Side, Twists, Forward, & Backward)
Basics Squat
Goblet Squat
Sandbag Squat
Resistance Band Squat
Squat and Row
Press and Squat
Balance Ball Squat
Dumbbell Squat
Medicine Ball Squat
Chair Squat
Medicine Ball Squat
Sumo Squat
Chair Pile Squat
Side-Leaning Sumo Squat
Toe-Touch Sumo Squat
Toe-Touch Sumo Squat
Medicine Ball Sumo Squat with Overhead Lift
Weighted Sumo Squat
Swiss Ball Wall Squat
Burpees
Supermans
Single Leg Deadlifts (with Dumbbells or without)
Step-Ups (Side, twists, Forward, & backward)
Step-Downs
Straight Kicks
Kick with Toe Touch
Kick with Arm Reach
Switch Kick Punch

Side Kick
Swiss Ball Side Kicks
Round Kick
Side Kick Punch
Round Kick
Lateral Bounding
Lateral Shuffle
Slalom Jumps
Swimming
Arm Hauler
Facedown Snow Angel
Superman
Supine Flutter Kicks
Diagonal Reach
Over-the-Shoulder Throw
Figure 8

Reflection Notes:

Reflection Notes – Continued:

Reflection Notes – Continued:

Reflection Notes – Continued:

Auxiliary

Lifting Terminology

Abduction: Movement of a limb away from the middle of the body.

Adduction: Movement of a limb towards the middle of the body.

Aerobic: An action or exercise that occurs or requires the presence of oxygen.

Agility: The ability to accelerate, decelerate, stabilize, and change direction quickly, while staying balanced and keeping good body posture.

Anaerobic: Physical activity that is performed in short, fast bursts ensuring that the heart cannot supply oxygen at a rate that the body needs.

Atrophy: A decrease in muscle size due to improper nutrition, or lack of exercise.

Barbell: A bar, usually 6-7 ft in length, in which weights are placed on both ends and used for resistance training.

Biomechanics: A study that uses principles of physics to quantitatively study how forces interact within a living body.

Body Composition: Breakdown of a body makeup, including body fat, lean muscle, and water.

Cardiorespiratory System: A system comprised of the cardiovascular and respiratory systems

Cardiovascular System: The system comprised of the heart, blood, and the blood vessels that transport the blood from the heart to the tissues of the body

Cardiovascular Endurance: The body's ability to gather, process, and deliver oxygen to the rest of the body.

Circuit Training: Performing multiple exercises (usually 2-4 different exercises) with little to no rest in between the different exercises.

Clean: Olympic style lift where weight is lifted from floor to shoulder in one movement including a catch phrase.

Clean and Jerk: Olympic style lift where weight is lifted from floor to overhead in two movements including a catch and press phase.

Concentric Muscle Action: Moving in the opposite direction of force, or the "pushing/pulling" part of a lift. Accelerates or produces force while contracting the muscle.

Controlled Instability: A training environment that is unstable, but can safely be controlled by an individual, in order to simulate a playing condition.

The Core: The lumbo-pelvic-hip and the thoracic and cervical spine, where the body's center of gravity is located.

Creatine Phosphate: A high-energy phosphate molecule that is stored in cells and can be used to resynthesize ATP immediately, during resistance training, or activities such as football, this is the body's primary energy source.

Deadlift: Weightlifting exercise where weight is lifted from floor to waist height, pressing with the legs and hinged hips, ending with back straight.

Decelerate: When the muscle is exerting less force than is being placed on it; or to reduce force.

Deconditioned: A state of lost physical fitness which includes muscle imbalances, decreased muscle flexibility, and a lack of core stability.

Dietary Supplement: A substance that completes or makes an addition to daily dietary intake, that is not meant to replace food or exercise, but instead compliments them.

Dorsiflexion: When applied to the ankle, it is the ability to bend at the ankle moving the front of the foot upward.

Dumbbell: Hand held weights that usually come in pairs ranging from 5-150 lbs.

Duration: The length of time something takes to happen.

Dynamic Functional Flexibility: Soft tissue extensibility with optimal neuromuscular efficiency throughout a full range of motion.

Dynamic Joint Stabilization: The stabilizing muscles that are a part of a joint to produce optimum stabilization during functional multiplanar movements.

Dynamic Range of Motion: The combination of flexibility and the nervous system's ability to control the range and movement.

Dynamic Stretching: Taking a joint through the full available range of motion using movement and force production.

Eccentric Muscle Action: The lengthening of the muscle to a resting length, or known as the negative phase of a lift (lowering the bar or weight during a push or pull exercise).

Equilibrium: the body's balance between opposite forces, influences or actions.

Exhaustion: Stress that causes the body to reach a level of depleted energy sources.

Extension: A body part going from a bent position to a straight position.

Fast Twitch Fibers: Muscle fibers that are often characterized by the term type IIA and type IIB. These fibers contain fewer capillaries mitochondria and myoglobin. These fibers fatigue faster than type one fibers or "slow twitch fibers".

Fatty Acids: Lipids used to create ATP while muscle cells are using aerobic energy systems. Oxygen must be present in order for muscle cells to convert fatty acids into ATP.

Fitness: A level in which a body can complete physical tasks. Different components of fitness include but are not limited to muscular strength, muscular endurance, flexibility, agility, power, strength, velocity, and more.

Flexibility: Having complete range of motion around a joint.

Flexion: The bending of a joint, causing the angle to the joint to decrease.

Frequency: How often something is completed.

General Warm-Up: A low intensity exercise consisting of movements that do not necessarily relate to the more intense exercise that is to follow.

Giant Set: Performing three exercises back to back to back with minimal rest in between.

Glycolysis: The metabolic pathway that converts glucose into ATP/energy.

Glycogen: Glucose stored in your muscles.

Ground Reaction Force: The equal and opposite force that is exerted back onto the body whenever the ground is touched with the body -- including steps, jumping, falling, etc.

Heart Rate Training Zones: Resting heart rate, target heart rate, maximum heart rate.

Hypertension: Blood pressure of 140/90 or higher

Hypertrophy: An increase in muscle size in response to overcoming force from high volumes of tension.

Intensity: The level to which a task is completed. How much weight, the tempo (how fast to complete exercise), or how many repetitions.

Isometric Muscle Action: No visible movement with or against resistance.

Isotonic Exercise: A type of exercise that results in the muscles lengthening or shortening while the tension remains the same. Free weight lifting is a form of isotonic exercise.

Joints: Where movements occur as a result of muscle contraction.

Lactic Acid: Produced during anaerobic exercise, contributes to fatigue.

Length: Tension Relationship: the length at which the muscles can produce the greatest force.

Linear Progression: Intensity or weight, either one or the other is incrementally increased every repeated workout to invoke the stress-recovery-adaptation response. The best way to practice this is to add to the max percentage for each week's lifts.

Maximal Strength: The maximum force that a muscle can produce in a voluntary single effort, regardless of the velocity.

Muscular Endurance: The ability of the body to produce force and maintain it for extended period of time

Muscular System: Controlled by the nervous system, these groups of musculus fibers manipulate and control the skeletal system of the human body.

Midline: Line that splits the body directly in half from left and right.

Muscle Fiber: There are many different types. These are the tiny fibers that construct a muscle of whatever group. Usually about 40 millimeters long.

Muscle Imbalance: Alteration of muscle length surrounding a joint.

Nervous System: A countless amount of cells forming nerves that are specifically designed to provide a communication network within the human body.

Neurotransmitter: Chemical messengers that cross synapses to transmit electrical impulses from the nerve to the muscle.

Nutrition: The sum of processes by which a living organism takes in and uses as food to fuel.

Obesity: Excessive amount of body fat (BMI = 30 or greater). Fastest growing health problem in the US.

Over Training: When an athlete is underperforming due to too much training and not enough recovery time. It is a physical and **psychological** problem.

Oxidation: The production of energy from the respiratory process in which you breathe in oxygen and that oxygen then "oxidizes" (or reacts with) fatty acids.

Pattern Overload: Doing the same exercise or workouts for too long of a time. Repeating the same pattern of movements.

Plyometrics: Also known as jump training or plyos. These are exercises in which muscles exert maximum force in short intervals of time, with the goal of increasing power (speed-strength).

Power: the ability to exert maximal force in the shortest amount of time. **(Force x Distance) / Time = Power**

Program Design: A purposeful system or plan created to enhance the ability of a group or individual in achieving a goal.

Protein: Amino acids linked by peptide bonds.

Quickness: The ability to react and change body position with maximum rate of force production.

Rate of Force Production: How quickly a muscle can generate force.

Reactive Strengths: The ability of the neuromuscular system to switch from eccentric contraction to a concentric contraction quickly and efficiently.

Reactive Training: Training techniques that use quick, powerful movements involving an eccentric contraction immediately followed an explosive concentric contraction.

Relative Flexibility: The tendency of the body to seek the path of least resistance during functional movement patterns

Repetition: The amount of times an athlete lifts and lowers the weight within a set.

Repetition Tempo: How fast or slow to move the weight during a rep.

Repetition Maximum: "MAX OUT" -- What is the maximum amount of weight that can be performed during a rep or a selected amount of reps.

Resistance: Acting against a force.

Respiratory System: The system of the body responsible for taking in oxygen, excreting carbon dioxide, and regulating the relative compositions of the blood.

Rest: Allowing recovery via time away from certain activity.

Rest Between Sets: This is the amount of time that you rest between each set to allow reoxygenation of the muscles. Usually between 1-3 minutes is ideal for most athletic training programs.

Set: How many times an athlete will perform a specific exercise. Example: Anthony will do 4 sets of squats 10 times each set. 4 sets X 10 reps

Slow Twitch Fibers: Another term for type one muscle fibers, fibers that are characterized by a greater amount of capillaries mitochondria and myoglobin. These fibers are found to have a higher level of endurance than those of fast twitch fibers.

Specific Warm-up: Pre competition exercise that allow the muscle to mimic sport specific movements at low to moderate intensity, allowing muscles to be properly activated.

Speed: the ability to move the body as fast as possible regardless of direction.

Spotter: A teammate, coach, or trainer that is aware of safety procedures and proper technique. This person's first job is to make sure that reps are completed safely, and with good technique. Each lift will usually have very specific actions the spotter must take in order to help the lifting athlete.

Strength: Force produced against an external resistance. Also known as work.

Stability: The ability of the body to maintain postural equilibrium and support joints during movements.

Superset: Two different exercises that are performed back to back without any rest time in-between them. They usually are contrasting exercises.

Supination/Pronation: Rotation of the foot or forearm so that the sole or palm face anteriorly (supination) or posteriorly (pronation). "Overhanded" grip is pronation. "Underhand" grip is supination.

Technique: A way of doing an activity that needs skill properly.

Tempo: The timing of the three phases of a rep—eccentric, amortization (or isometric), and concentric.

Tendon: Attaches muscle to bone.

Training Intensity: An individual's level of effort, compared with their maximum effort, which is usually expressed as a percentage.

Vo2 Max: The highest rate of oxygen transport and utilization achieved at maximal physical exertion.

Volume: "How much" -- Hypotrophy phases will be the highest volume during a periodized program, it will consist of the most amount of reps and sets. The Power Phase will consist of the lowest volume, low reps, and sets with high intensity.

Abbreviated Lifting Terminology

AMRAP = As many reps as possible
AS = Assisted
BB = Barbell
BP = Bench Press
BW = Body Weight
C2B = Chest to Bar, as in chest to bar pull-ups
CB = Cable
C&J = Clean and jerk
CG = Close Grip
COD = Cut on a Dime
CT = Circuit Training
DB = Dumbbell
DL = Deadlift
DOMS = Delayed Onset Muscle Soreness
Ex = Exercise
ExRx = Exercise Prescription
FSQ = Front Squat
GHD = Glute Ham Developer
GHR = Glute ham raise
HIT = High Intense Training
HSPU = Hand stand push up
IBP = Incline Bench Press
KB = Kettlebell
KBS = Kettlebell Swing
LV = Lever
Hang (as in "hang clean") = The lift starts with the bar being deadlifted to the hip, then lowered to the appropriate hang position.

Abbreviated Lifting Terminology -- Continued

Metcon = A workout focused on metabolic conditioning.
MU = Muscle ups.
OHP = Overhead Press
OHS = Overhead squat.
OHSQ = Overhead Squat
MP = Military Press
NG = Narrow Grip
PR = Personal Record
R = Resistance
R90, R60… = Rest 90 seconds
RDL = Romanian Deadlift
Rep = Repetition. One performance of an exercise.
RM = Repetition maximum. Your 1RM is your max lift for one rep. Your 10 RM is the most you can lift 10 times.
ROM = Range of Motion
Set = A number of repetitions. e.g., 3 sets of 10 reps, often seen as 3×10, means do 10 reps, rest, repeat, rest, repeat.
SLDL = Stiff or Straight Legged Deadlifts
SM = Smith Machine
SL = Sled
SQ = Squat
TNG = Touch and Go- the transition from each rep to the next should be quick, basically "touching" the bar to the floor and immediately going into next rep
T2B = Toes to bar
TUT = Time under Tension
WOD = Workout of the day
WG = Wide Grip
WT = Weight or Weight

Neck Stretches

Coaching Tip: It is very important to keep the body and shoulders straight and level.

Disclaimer: Please discuss stretching in more detail with your Athletic Trainer or Team Doctor. I am a firm believer in having players stretch their necks to help maintain the overall well being of their body before a practice or game. Always take physical restrictions into consideration before advising a player to do a specific stretch or drill. I am not a doctor and I do not assume responsibility. I am just sharing effective ways to stretch a specific area. Please understand the stretches thoroughly and give proper instruction when directing players.

Individual Stretching:

1) Roll your head/neck clockwise and count to 10.

2) Roll your head/neck counter-clockwise and count to 10.

3) Look to your left, hold that position, and count to 10.

4) Look to your right, hold that position, and count to 10.

Individual Stretching – Adding Resistance:

1) Place your left palm on the right side of your head and gently pull toward your left shoulder – count to 10.

2) Place your right palm on the left side of your head and gently pull toward your right shoulder – count to 10.

Partner Stretching – Adding Resistance:

- **NOTE:** Player #1 is getting stretched while wearing a helmet, and Player #2 is adding the resistance to the stretch.

Coaching Tip: Make sure that Player #1 knows not to push too hard – this is just for slight resistance stretching and that Player #2 does not push back, they are only there to provide resistance.

1) Player #1 is in a 6-point stance where the hands, knees and toes are on the ground. Player #2 is standing to one side of Player #1. While Player #1 is on the ground, Player #2's leg will stand firm to provide resistance as Player #1 slightly pushes their head against Player #2's leg and counts to 10.

2) Same as step 1 but have Player #2 switch sides.

3) Player #1 is in a 6-point stance where the hands, knees and toes are on the ground. Player #2 is standing in front of Player #1 so Player #1's head is at Player #2's knees. Player #2 places both hands so they barely touch the back of Player #1's helmet. Player #1 slightly pushes their head up against Player #2's hands and counts to 10.

4) Player #1 is in a 6-point stance where the hands, knees and toes are on the ground. Player #2 is standing in front of Player #1 so Player #1's head is at Player #2's knees. Player #2 places both hands so they gently cradle the front of Player #1's face mask. Player #1 slightly pushes their head down against Player #2's hands and counts to 10.

5) Player #1 and Player #2 switch roles so Player #2 completes steps 1-4.

Walking

This is one exercise that is definitely overlooked by a lot of people. It is important to start somewhere simple yet effective especially if you are helping a person that is overweight. They can't just start a normal athletic routine. The big thing is having a watch that tracks your movement or a phone with an app that you carry to track how much you actually move. A lot of people say that anywhere from 5,000 to 15,000 steps is a good number to average on a daily or weekly basis. Aim high. A weekly average of 15,000+ steps during the work week is great and then anywhere from 10,000+ is good because a lot of us probably don't have their phone on them 100% of the time to track their steps. Since the start of Covid-19, there has been a huge increase in people walking outside. Walking has a lot of benefits -- here are just a few:

1) Improves circulation
2) Walking 30+ minutes a day can help improve bone mass
3) You will live longer
4) It helps with anger issues / relieve stress
5) Lose weight -- but you have to do it over 30 minutes or more
6) Helps maintain healthy muscles & joints
7) Improves sleeping -- especially when you get older
8) Improves breathing

Walking will help with a lot of things, but just like everything in this book, start slow and build up to 30 minutes or longer.

Coaching Tip: Make sure you have a good pair of tennis shoes with proper support.

Yoga

Disclaimer: Please discuss stretching, such as Yoga, in more detail with your Athletic Trainer or Team Doctor. We are firm believers in having players stretch their muscles to help maintain the overall well being of their body before a practice or game. Always take physical restrictions into consideration before advising a player to do a specific stretch or drill. We are not doctors and do not assume responsibility. We are just sharing effective ways to stretch a specific area. Please understand the stretches thoroughly and give proper instruction when directing players.

Reasons why to have your players do YOGA:

1) It improves their posture
2) It will improve their overall flexibility
3) It can reduce the risk of injury – Different Yoga poses target specific muscles
4) Increases concentration
5) Gain strength and stamina
6) Improves balance and stability
7) Develops better body awareness

Coach Stone first started doing DDP YOGA© around five years ago, yes, the wrestler. It is actually a very good regiment and comes with its own workout plan, DVD, and now there is an app out for it.

We have listed a few Yoga poses that you can have your players do at school, their house, or wherever you work out as a team. Look the poses up on the Internet and share videos with players to create your own workout regimen.

Consider investing in the following items to help make Yoga more effective:

1) Yoga Mat (or beach towel)
2) Water (a lot)
3) Clean Feet (especially if you do it with more people)
4) Towel (to wipe sweat away)

Yoga is mild but very effective. You can do Yoga everyday within reason, but don't overdo it. (Refer to the disclaimer above.)

Recommendation: Do Yoga anywhere from 20 minutes to 1 hour everyday – but no longer than that.

Start small with the following six poses listed below.

1) Standing
2) Front Bends
3) Back Bends
4) Arm Movements
5) Seated Poses
6) Sprawl Poses

Coaching Tip: Make up a Yoga routine that works for you or look into DDP YOGA©.

Standing - These poses are considered the foundation of YOGA.

Here are just a few you can do – no certain order:

* These are not for Beginners

Mountain Pose	Upward Salute	Reverse Prayer*	Hands Bound	Sideways Hands Bound	Standing Crescent
Tadasana Pose	One Leg Standing Crescent	Sun Salutation BackBend *	Chair Pose	Tree Pose	Tree Pose with Side Bending*
Arms Raised	Extended Hand to Foot Pose	Leg to Side	Upward Extended *	Triangle Pose	Revolved Triangle Pose*
Extended Side Triangle*	Warrior Pose	Tiptoe Warrior	Extended Side Angle Pose		

Forward Bends - These are the poses that create space and length in the spine. It also strengthens the lower parts of the body like: hamstrings, calves, hips, knees, and thighs.

Here are just a few you can do – no certain order:

* These are not for Beginners

Intense Side Stretch Preparation	Intense Side Stretch Hands to Foot	Intense Side Stretch Hands to Leg*	Intense Side Stretch Forehead to Shin*
Standing Forward Bend	Wide Legged Forward Bend*	Half Feet Out	Half Feet Out Backhand*
Seated Forward Bend	Hands over Heels	Hands to Ground	Child's Pose
Child's Pose with Extended Arms	Child's Pose Hands to the Side	Child's Pose Palms Together	Extended Puppy Pose
Bound Angle Pose	Bound Angle Pose with Hands in Prayer	Fire Log Pose	Wide Angle Seated Bend*

Back Bends - These poses are the backbone of Yoga. Make sure you don't move too fast while doing these poses.

Here are just a few you can do – no certain order:

* These are not for Beginners

Upward Facing Dog	Upward Facing Dog Extended	Raised Hips Extended	Upward Facing Dog Tiptoes*
Cobra	Half Frog Pose*	Bow Pose*	Bridge Pose
Bridge Pose Preparation	Bridge Hands to Back	Bridge Arms Overhead	Bridge Hands to Ankle*
Upward Facing Bow Pose	Camel Pose*	Fish Pose*	Locust Pose*

Arm Movements - These poses help strength the upper body, specifically the arms, shoulders, and chest.

Here are just a few you can do – no certain order:

* These are not for Beginners

Plank Pose	Plank Pose Preparation	One Handed Extended Four Limbed Staff Pose	One Leg Staff Pose
Staff Pose Revolved One Hand	Chaturanga	Side Plank	Downward Facing Dog
Plow Pose	Shoulder Stand	Leg Contraction Pose	Upward Facing Plank
Feet Wide Eastern Intense Stretch	Eastern Intense Stretch Pose		

Seated - These poses help strengthen and improve range of motion, in addition to releasing any tension you might have.

Here are just a few you can do – no certain order:

* These are not for Beginners

Staff Pose	Staff Pose Heart to Sky	Easy Pose	Easy Pose on Block
Accomplished Pose	Hero Pose	Tiptoe Hero Pose	Hero Pose Dog Tilt Backbend
Hero Pose Raised Bound Hands	Full Lotus Pose*	Half Lotus Pose*	Lotus with Upward-Bound Hands*
Boat Pose	Easy Boat Pose	Easy Boat Pose Crunch	Sage Marichi's Pose
Monkey Pose*			

Sprawl - These poses would be considered part of a cooldown in Yoga while helping with hips, lower legs, and back support.

Here are just a few you can do – no certain order:

* These are not for Beginners

Reclining Twist	Knees to Chest Pose	One Legged Wind Relieving Pose	Reclining Tree Pose*
Corpse Pose	Reclining Legs Extended Pose		

Weight-Less 2-Week Program

As unfortunate as it is, we do understand that not every program has access to a weight room, and during the COVID-19 Pandemic, weight room access is often limited, or restricted. However, it is possible to create a conditioning program that is not limited to your resources. This allows you to help your athletes keep their bodies ready so they can be successful and healthy.

The following is the 2-Week Program that Coach Casazza used with his players during the start of the pandemic. His players continued to cycle through the 2-Week Program until the team was able to meet in-person again.

Conditioning Progression

Week 1-

SKILLS-

Monday

- 6x 50-yard Sprints (30 seconds Rest)
- 40 Push-Ups / 40 Body Squats

Tuesday

- 5x 60-yard Shuttles
- 50 Sit-Ups / 75 Supermans

Thursday

- 6x 20-yard Backpedals Flip Hip 20-yard Sprint (30 seconds rest)
- 50 Push-Ups / 50 Body Squats

MIDS-

Monday

- 6x 40-yard Sprints (30 seconds Rest)
- 50 Push-Ups / 50 Body Squats

Tuesday

- 5x 60-yard Shuttles
- 50 Sit-Ups / 75 Supermans

Thursday

- 8 Hill Sprints (30 seconds rest)
- 60 Push-Ups / 60 Body Squats

BIGS-

Monday

- 6x 30-yard Sprints (30 seconds Rest)
- 50 Push-Ups / 50 Body Squats

Tuesday

- 5x 45-yard Shuttles
- 50 Sit-Ups/ 75 Supermans

Thursday

- 6 Hill Sprints (30 seconds rest)
- 60 Push-Ups / 60 Body Squats

Week 2-

SKILLS-

Monday

- 10x 50-yard Sprints (30 seconds Rest)
- 60 Push-Ups / 60 Body Squats
- Shoulder Circuit 2x 30sec each
  * Palm Down Flutter
  * Palm Out Flutter
  * Palm Back
  * Pronate-Supinate
  * Raise the Roof

Tuesday

- 8x 60-yard Shuttles
- 100 Sit-Ups / 100 Supermans
- Bulldog Circuit 2x 10 each way
  * Fire Hydrant
  * Forward Circles
  * Backward Circles
  * Leg Out Raises

Wednesday

- 3x 30-yard Broad Jumps
- 3x 50 Squat Jumps
- 3x 20 each Leg Split Squat Jumps
- 3x 20 each Leg Ski Jumps
- 5x 40-yard Sprints (position specific stance)

Thursday

- 10x 20-yard Backpedals Flip Hip 20-yard Sprint (30 seconds rest)
- 75 Push-Ups / 75 Body Squats
- 3x 1 min. each Plank Circuit
    * Normal
    * Left Side
    * Right Side

MIDS-

Monday

- 10x 40-yard Sprints (30 seconds Rest)
- 75 Push-Ups / 75 Body Squats
- Shoulder Circuit 2x 30sec each
    * Palm Down Flutter
    * Palm Out Flutter
    * Palm Back
    * Pronate-Supinate
    * Raise the Roof

Tuesday

- 5x 60-yard Shuttles
- 100 Sit-Ups / 100 Supermans
- Bulldog Circuit 2x 10 each way
    * Fire Hydrant
    * Forward Circles
    * Backward Circles
    * Leg Out Raise
    * Donkey Kicks

Wednesday

- 3x 30-Yard Broad Jumps
- 3x 50 Squat Jumps
- 3x 20 each Leg Split Squat Jumps
- 3x 20 each Leg Ski Jumps
- 5x 40-yard Sprints (position specific stance)

Thursday

- 12 Hill Sprints (30 seconds rest)
- 100 Push-Ups / 100 Body Squats
- 3x 1 min. Each Plank Circuit
    * Normal
    * Left Side
    * Right Side

BIGS-

Monday

- 10x 40-yard Sprints (30 seconds Rest)
- 75 Push-Ups / 75 Body Squats
- Shoulder Circuit 2x 30sec each
    * Palm Down Flutter
    * Palm Out Flutter
    * Palm Back
    * Pronate-Supinate
    * Raise the Roof

Tuesday

- 8x 45-yard Shuttles
- 80 Sit-Ups / 80 Supermans
- Bulldog Circuit 2x 10 each way
    * Fire Hydrant
    * Forward Circles
    * Backward Circles
    * Leg Out Raise
    * Donkey Kicks

Wednesday

- 3x 30-yard Broad Jumps
- 3x 50 Squat Jumps
- 3x 20 each Leg Split Squat Jumps
- 3x 20 each Leg Ski Jumps
- 5x 40-yard Sprints (position specific stance)

Thursday

- 10 Hill Sprints (30 seconds rest)
- 100 Push-Ups / 100 Body Squats
- 3x 1 min. each Plank Circuit
    * Normal
    * Left Side
    * Right Side

Nutrition Tips & Tricks

Disclaimer: Consult with your Dietitian or Doctor before dieting or changing your eating habits. We are firm believers in eating correctly to help maintain the overall well-being of our bodies. We are not doctors and we do not assume responsibility for your decisions. The following is an example of possible effective ways to eat right with a person that weighs 180 pounds.

EXAMPLE NUTRITION GUIDE
MEAL / EATING GUIDE

WEIGHT- 180 LBS
GOAL- ATTAIN A HEALTHY WEIGHT

Player 1 will need to up their Calories by 12%-15%
2,500cal x 15% (12-15%) = 375 cals. 2,500 cal + 375
= 2,875 cals daily.

To lose weight at a healthy rate, take 8-10 calories and multiply it by every pound of body weight. Example 320 lbs x 9 cals = 2,880 cals daily. From there, you can break down macronutrients from the following example below.

To maintain weight, take 10-12 calories and multiply it by every pound of body weight. 250 lbs x 11 cals = 2,750 cals daily.

We are only using 2,500 cals as an example for a reference point. This does not mean it is a set calorie intake number and often time may not be the case. A lot of the times it will be more, and in some cases it will be less.

- To build and develop healthy muscles, the athlete will need to consume 2,500-2,900 cals daily.

Protein: 1 Gram Protein = 4 Calories
Carbs: 1 Gram Carbs = 4 Calories
Fat: 1 Gram Fat = 9 Calories

***Protein:** Protein will need to be the first thing calculated, the calculation is 1.2 grams of protein per pound of CURRENT body weight. (We are still using our example of a 180 lbs)

- **EXAMPLE:** 180 lbs x 1.2 = **216 Grams of Protein**
  216 Grams x 4 cal per grams of Protein = 864 Protein Cal

***Fat:** Fat should range between 25-30% of your total Calories. This is the most calorie dense macronutrient.

- **Example:** 2,875 Total cal x 30% = **863 Fat Calories**
  863 Fat cal / 9 cal = **95 Grams of Fat**

Carbs: It is really simple to figure out the amount of carbohydrates needed. Just add the left-over Protein and Fat calories together and the remaining amount will be the Carbohydrate intake.

- **Example:**
  864 (Protein Calories) + 863 (Fat Calories) = 1,727 Cal
  2,875 (Total Calories) - 1,727 (Protein & Fat Cal) = 1,148 Cal
  1,148 Cal / 4 cal per gram of Carbs
  = **287 grams of Carbs daily**

The following are recommended food groups, and more specifically what to choose from:

CARBS:

Brown rice - Sweet potatoes - Oats - Quinoa - Bread - Apples & Oranges - Majority of fruits & vegetables - Whole wheat bread - Pinto beans - Squash, Pasta, Potatoes (try to avoid anything fried).

PROTEINS:

Chicken (try to avoid breaded and fried) - Turkey breast - Beef - Bison - Salmon - Fish (try to avoid breaded and fried) - Cottage cheese.

FATS:

Olive oil - MCT oil - Avocado - Grape seed oil, avocado oil - Almonds, cashews, sunflower seeds, pumpkin seeds - peanuts - peanut butter - Fish oil Supplements - Fats from meats (salmon, beef, pork all have a high good fat content.)

FRUITS:

Grapefruit - Watermelon - Strawberries - Blackberries - Oranges - Cantaloupe – Banana – Raspberries – Grapes – Apples, etc.

VEGETABLES:

Carrots - Brussel sprouts - Green beans - Broccoli - Asparagus - Cauliflower - onions, bell peppers, etc.

DIARY:

Milk - Chocolate Milk.

SUMMARY:

(Daily Calorie intake is based on our example weight of 180 lbs.)

⇒ EAT 2,500-2,875 CALORIES DAILY FOR HEALTHY WEIGHT GAIN

⇒ FOLLOW THE ABOVE FOOD LIST FOR RECOMMENDED FOODS

Coaching Tip: ALWAYS CARRY A JAR OF PEANUT BUTTER (OR THE TO-GO CUPS) WITH YOU AT SCHOOL OR ON WHEN YOU ARE ON THE GO AND EAT A SPOONFUL EVERY 1-2 HOURS.

ALWAYS BE EATING!!!!!!!!

Our bodies respond well to consistency: wake up and go to bed at the same time, eat at the same time, exercise/physical activity on a daily basis, etc. Find a routine that works for you and watch what an overall difference it makes and how much better you will feel.

Coaching Tip: Eat small, frequent meals/snacks (like every 2-3 hours) rather than 2-3 large meals a day.

OFFSEASON PROGRAM TEMPLATE©

WEEK 1 HYPERTROPHY	DAY	EXERCISE -POWER -STRENGTH -AUX LIFTS	SETS/REPS	INTENSITY	WEIGHT USED

WEEK 2 HYPERTROPHY	DAY	EXERCISE -POWER -STRENGTH -AUX LIFTS	SETS/REPS	INTENSITY	WEIGHT USED

WEEK 3 HYPERTROPHY	DAY	EXERCISE -POWER -STRENGTH -AUX LIFTS	SETS/REPS	INTENSITY	WEIGHT USED

WEEK 4 HYPERTROPHY	DAY	EXERCISE -POWER -STRENGTH -AUX LIFTS	SETS/REPS	INTENSITY	WEIGHT USED

WEEK 5 BASIC STRENGTH	DAY	EXERCISE -POWER -STRENGTH -AUX LIFTS	SETS/REPS	INTENSITY	WEIGHT USED

WEEK 6 BASIC STRENGTH	DAY	EXERCISE -POWER -STRENGTH -AUX LIFTS	SETS/REPS	INTENSITY	WEIGHT USED

WEEK 7 BASIC STRENGTH	DAY	EXERCISE -POWER -STRENGTH -AUX LIFTS	SETS/REPS	INTENSITY	WEIGHT USED

WEEK 8 BASIC STRENGTH	DAY	EXERCISE -POWER -STRENGTH -AUX LIFTS	SETS/REPS	INTENSITY	WEIGHT USED

WEEK 9 POWER	DAY	EXERCISE -POWER -STRENGTH -AUX LIFTS	SETS/REPS	INTENSITY	WEIGHT USED

WEEK 10 POWER	DAY	EXERCISE -POWER -STRENGTH -AUX LIFTS	SETS/REPS	INTENSITY	WEIGHT USED

WEEK 11 POWER	DAY	EXERCISE -POWER -STRENGTH -AUX LIFTS	SETS/REPS	INTENSITY	WEIGHT USED

WEEK 12 POWER	DAY	EXERCISE -POWER -STRENGTH -AUX LIFTS	SETS/REPS	INTENSITY	WEIGHT USED

WEEKs 13-16 PEAK/ MAINTENANCE	DAY	EXERCISE -POWER -STRENGTH -AUX LIFTS	SETS/REPS	INTENSITY	WEIGHT USED

Football Resources
By Coach Stone

I highly recommend visiting my website www.CoachStoneFootball.com for direct links to amazing football resources. I am a firm believer in each of the companies listed on my website and I believe they can help every team and organization in more ways than one. Be sure to use my special promo codes for each located on the bottom of my website or next to each of their logos.

I

Football Resources -- Continued

Alphabetical Order:

- ✓ 2nd Skull® (Promo Code)
- ✓ 3Dimensional Coaching™
- ✓ Atavus (Promo Code)
- ✓ Athlete Intelligence
- ✓ DragonFly Athletics
- ✓ Fantom Athletics (Promo Code)
- ✓ FNF Coaches (Promo Code)
- ✓ GoArmy Edge Football
- ✓ Guardian Caps (Refer Coach Stone for discount)
- ✓ HIGHandTIGHT (Promo Code)
- ✓ Just Play Solutions (Promo Code)
- ✓ Knack Bags (https://knackbags.com)
- ✓ Launch Pad Kickoff Tee (Promo Code)
- ✓ P2Bar
- ✓ PB Athletics (Promo Code)
- ✓ S.A.F.E.Clip (Promo Code)
- ✓ Sadler Sports & Recreation Insurance
- ✓ TackleBar™
- ✓ Tackle Tube USA™ (Promo Code)
- ✓ Turk Tank (Promo Code)
- ✓ WatchGameFilm (Promo Code)

About the Authors

Coach Anthony Stone grew up in Hometown, Illinois with his parents (Carol and William) and older brother (Bill). He went to Hometown Elementary School where his passion for all sports was born. Growing up he played football, baseball, basketball, and wrestling. He knew at a young age that he wanted to be an NFL player or a teacher. Sports gave him the desire to pursue his education. He went on to complete his B.A. in Physical Education (K-6th and 7-12th teaching certificate and coaching certification.) He was never able to get into the NFL but he was fortunate enough to try out for the Chicago Rush (AFL) twice in 2001 and 2002. Later, with the support of his wife, Kara Stone, he signed an indoor football contract with the Rock River Raptors (UIF) in 2006 as a quarterback. If it wasn't for his physical education teachers and coaches pushing him to always be a leader, he probably wouldn't be writing these books today.

After completing his M.A.T. in Special Education in 2001, he went on to work for two private schools in the Rockford area. He created both of their physical education programs and incorporated *The Big 4: Physical Education* (his first book) to complement his lessons. His second book, *Back to the Basics: Football Drill Manual* is filled with over 500+ pages of football content. There are 20 total Volumes scheduled to be published that build on the content found in the original *Football Drill Manual*. Stone has been teaching for over 15 years in the Rockford area. He has invented numerous games that were inspired by interactions with his own children during the summer months.

Coach Anthony Stone has been presenting at Physical Education Conventions for over 6 years in two different states. He has also published over 50 blogs on football and how to teach sports.

Anthony spends his spare time running his company, Coach Stone Football. His customizable football camp is available for youth, tackle and professional organizations of every level in every country. The purpose of his camp is to instill confidence in athletes by laying a foundation. His football camp, Back to the Basics, specializes in player camps, Coaches Clinics: X's & O's, Moms of Football Clinic: Fan to Team Mom to Coach, film evaluation, and more. When he's not teaching, traveling, or coaching he is enjoying life with his beautiful wife Kara and their five children.

You can reach Coach Stone via email at CoachStoneUSA@gmail.com or by visiting his website at www.CoachStoneFootball.com.

Coach Stone's Tip:
Go to www.CoachStoneFootball.com for special discount codes under the Sponsor Section.

Follow him on Twitter: @Coach_Stone_MT
Subscribe to his YouTube Channel: Coach Stone Football: Back to the Basics

Coach Cody Casazza grew up in Rockford, Illinois. Growing up, sports would eventually become the focal point of everyday life, having played baseball, basketball, and football both organized and recreational at the parks with friends. For Casazza, football would not come until later in high school when he was approached to play by one Anthony Stone. That decision would become the center point for which would be the deciding factor in how Coach Casazza continues to spend his life. From the first day out on the field with teammates, to this very day, football has been everything. It is what led to him going to college at Rockford University earning his B.S in Physical education/ Exercise Science, then later his M. Ed in Instruction and Curriculum, and now earning National Certification from the National Council on Strength and Fitness as a Certified Strength Coach. Currently Coach Casazza Lives in Middle Tennessee, where he coaches Varsity Football, and is serving as the Strength and Conditioning Coordinator.

Follow him on Twitter: @CodyCasazza92
Subscribe to his YouTube Channel: Coach Casazza Strength & Conditioning

The following books are currently available to purchase:

- *The Big 4: Physical Education*
- *Back to the Basics: Football Drill Manual*
- *Back to the Basics: Football Drill Manual: Volume I Offense*
- *Back to the Basics: Football Drill Manual: Volume II Defense*
- *Back to the Basics: Football Drill Manual: Volume III Special Teams*
- *Back to the Basics: Football Drill Manual: Volume IV Tackling & Turnovers*
- *Back to the Basics: Football Drill Manual: Flag Football Edition*
- *Back to the Basics: Football Drill Manual: TackleBar™ Edition*
- *Back to the Basics: Football Clinic Notebook*
- *Back to the Basics: Skill Manual: Junior Sports (Co-Authors: Coach Anthony Stone & Coach Ricky Upton)*
- *Back to the Basics Football Manual: Moms Edition*
- *Back to the Basics: Football Drill Manual: Volume V Coaching Edition*
- *Back to the Basics: Daily Motivational Quotes*
- *Back to the Basics: DIY Football Drill Manual Notebook*
- *Back to the Basics: DIY Football Drill Manual Booklet*
- *Back to the Basics: DIY Football Playbook*

- *Back to the Basics: DIY Flag Football Playbook*
- *Back to the Basics: Strength & Conditioning Manual (Co-Authors: Coach Anthony Stone & Coach Cody Casazza)*

Coming Soon:

- *Back to the Basics: Football Drill Manual: Volume VI Coaching Secrets*
- *Back to the Basics: Daily Motivational Quotes 2nd Edition*

Thank You

As a thank you for buying our book, Coach Stone will send you the editable versions of any of the Diagrams or Checklists in this book if you complete the following steps:

1) Post a picture of you holding this book on one of the following social media sites and use hashtag #BacktotheBasicsSC. If you do not have a social media account then send the pictures to Coach Stone so he can post it:

   Twitter: @Coach_Stone_MT
   Facebook: Anthony Stone (Coach Stone)
   Instagram: coach_stone_football
   Email: CoachStoneUSA@gmail.com

2) Write a review on Amazon.com.

Good luck with your upcoming season and thank you for choosing to go Back to the Basics,

Coach Anthony Stone
"Laying a foundation one drill at a time."

Coach Cody Casazza, NCSF

Printed in Great Britain
by Amazon

40317605R00123